S F NERV S

Safe, Inexpensive, Effective and Science Based Remedies for
Nerve Related Health Challenges

- Nerve Pain • Numbness
Needles • Nerve Damage
- Peripheral Neuropathy
- Facial Pain/Bells Palsy
  - Stabbing Feeling

- Tingling • Burning • Pins &
  - Electric Feelings • Cramps
  - Sciatica • Carpal Tunnel
  - Shingles • Neuralgia
  - Weakness & Stiffness

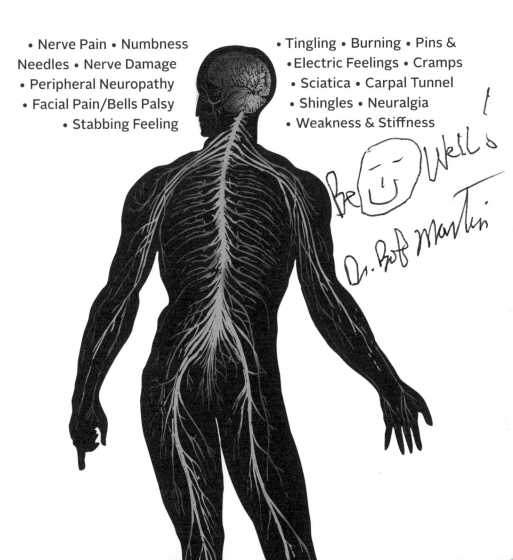

Be 🙂 Well !
Dr. Bob Martin

DR. BOB MARTIN

Host of America's #1 Nationally Syndicated
Health & Wellness Talk Show

For additional copies of this book visit www.doctorbob.com or call Better
Health Network at 1-808-322-2394.

No information contained herein is meant to replace the advice of a doctor
or healthcare practitioner. The data and opinions appearing in this book are
for informational purposes only. Readers are encouraged to seek advice from
qualified health professionals.

ISBN 978-193663104-9

Dedication

John and Frances Martin

I'm blessed to have had parents love me so deeply, encourage me so strongly and believe in me so very much.

AND

To my loving wife and six beautifully gifted children – if not for you my life would be incomplete.

Acknowledgements

It's been an honor to serve the many special people I've had the distinct privilege to care for as patients. Through our collective tribulations, victories and experiences together this book was made possible.

I am also grateful to the hundreds of thousands of dedicated and enthusiastic listeners of my weekly radio talk shows. Your desire to learn more about the subjects of health and wellness, challenges me to continue to seek out and deliver important information so as to help you become your own best doctor most of the time.

To the many health experts, providers and caregivers who chose to graciously take time out of their busy schedules to appear as guests on my radio talk show.

And to my many radio talk show sponsors who choose to support my efforts to help the sick and infirm find their way to health naturally, I am humbled by your generosity and commitment.

My appreciation and respect goes out to the many instructors and teachers I've studied under throughout my life. Their patience and dedication allowed me to realize my true calling.

Thank you to Darrin Cameron for his technical expertise as my behind the scenes radio show co-pilot and for his unwavering loyalty for nearly two decades. Thanks also to Irwin Zucker of Promotion in Motion for encouraging me to write a book every single time I run into him at conventions.

My colleagues and friends for their kindness and support including: Dr. Everett Beyer, Travis Anderson, Dr. Dan Crider, Dr. Chester Wilk, Dr. Ken Brockman, Dr. Clif Arrington, Dr, Juanee Surprise, Dr. Jodi Judge, Dr. David McCallan, Carl Gardner, Dan Deeb, Laurie Cantillo, Kevin Nitsche, Mike Taylor, Barry Young, Kim Komando, Smokey Rivers, Sue Swenson, Stuart Tomc, Stu Ferguson, Dr. Tony O'Donnell, Catie Noris, Dr. Richard Gingras, Dr. Greg Perea, Dr. Boris Schwartz, Dr. Russell Shurtleff, Dr. Robert Seamon, Dr. Chester Graham, Dr Bruce Shelton

For their skillful assistance and guidance in writing this book, I thank Emily Freeman, Cord Udall and McKinley Oswald.

Contents

Preface

As I entered into the my senior year of high school nearly four decades ago, my dad had the nerve to inform me that if I didn't intend on attending college in order to further my education, I would either have to pay for room and board while living under his roof or find somewhere else to live. Because my older brother, Dr. Brian Martin, was already attending college, the pressure to educate or vacate was very apparent.

I grew up in the Midwest and, being completely dependent on my parents, had no forethought, desire or intentions of moving anywhere – let along out into the cold cruel world on my own. My only real goal in life was to get out of school as quickly as possible and never go back. I figured I'd get a full-time job, earn some money, take a trip or two and eventually become confident enough to share an apartment with a friend or hopefully get married someday. However, I knew it would be very difficult to find a mate. That person would have to be willing to put up with all of my illnesses, take care of me as well as my mother had, and then, be my wife.

My entire childhood was filled with combinations of chronic illnesses including asthma, bronchitis, pneumonia, allergies, sinusitis, eczema, headaches and a supposed form of ADHD. This created a feeling of low self-confidence. Additionally, I was extremely shy and non-communicative with most people with the exception of family and close friends.

At around age fifteen, I became interested in girls and various forms of transportation including motorized mini bikes and cars. However, my dad believed that in order to enjoy the privilege of having one's own wheels, one would be required to fund the purchase of such luxuries. Therefore, I decided to get a part-time job in order to save up enough money to purchase a car. My older sister, Mollie Kling, helped me get a job at a local grocery store where she was working. I wasn't eligible to work since I hadn't yet turned sixteen but her boss was kind enough to allow me to work in the back of the grocery store –out of sight from any customers or labor inspectors.

Over the next year, I struggled to make it to school and to work due to the fact that I was often ill with any number of the sicknesses that seemed to plague me. I felt helpless, as I truly wanted to work in order to save up for a car purchase and attend high school in order to graduate on time.

One afternoon at work, a co-worker who stocked shelves asked me why I had to constantly blow my nose, sneeze and cough. My reply was, essentially, that it was a way of life for me and had been for the last fifteen years —or for as long as I could remember. He proceeded to explain that it wasn't normal to be sick all the time. He asked about the type of healthcare I was receiving. I went on to explain that I was taking multiple prescription drugs for my various symptoms. His next comment was, "It sure doesn't seem like it's doing much good for you."

Turns out that the shelf stocker was also a fulltime student at Palmer Chiropractic College in Davenport, Iowa. Over the next several weeks we talked whenever we saw each other in the company break room. Our conversations always seemed to revolve around his interest in my health or rather, the lack there-of.

I was complaining about having a headache at work one day and the chiropractic student explained that many headaches are caused by neck vertebrae or bone misalignments. In fact, he stated that many of the health concerns I suffered with could also be caused or made worse by spinal misalignments in my neck or back areas. Next, he offered to perform a brief evaluation of my neck and back areas on two gigantic boxes of Charmin toilet paper, which served as a makeshift exam bench. The impromptu exam was to take place in the rear of the store and out of sight of store customers and our boss. Being the naïve person I was at the time, I agreed to have him do an evaluation on my spine. He found several sore spots at the top of my neck area, and explained that I had spinal misalignments. It was his belief that the problems he found with my spine could be causing my current headache and possibly even other health concerns. He offered to do a Chiropractic adjustment of my neck.

Seconds later, he gently turned my head to the left and a large cracking noise emitted, then to the right with the same outcome. At first, I was scared that he had injured or broken my neck. But I quickly realized that I felt no pain and could still move my legs and arms. Once he finished with his treatment, I got off the big boxes full of toilet paper and stood-up. I felt different at first, as though someone had lifted a weight off my head. But, my headache was seventy five percent better and my neck felt much less tight.

Over the next several months, I received regular chiropractic adjustments whenever possible atop the toilet paper exam table. Over time, a most gratifying transformation of my health started to occur including having less sinus congestion, coughing, sneezing, and wheezing. Instead I felt a general sense of wellbeing.

My parents started to notice that I generally looked better, my appetite improved and I didn't require the frequent trips to the medical doctor for additional prescription drugs and antibiotic shots. Over the next six months I steadily got stronger and healthier.

One day the student asked me what I intend to do upon graduation from high school. I stated that I planned to get a job at one of the local factories. He reminded me of how much better I was feeling, functioning and performing, and suggested since I had such a strong response to chiropractic adjustments, I should consider becoming a doctor of chiropractic. I chuckled and replied, "Go to college? – I'm barely making it through high school due to my frequent absenteeism due to chronic illnesses." He offered to set up an appointment with the chiropractic college registrar, and I agreed. The registrar listened to the story about how my health had dramatically improved as a result of receiving chiropractic care. He explained that prior to professional college acceptance, I would be required to complete, a standard number of prerequisite college credits. I went on to complete the required college credits, got accepted into Chiropractic College and graduated four years later.

Upon graduating from Palmer College of Chiropractic, I started a practice in Denver, Colorado. After six months in practice the hard financial times started to get better as more patients found their way to my office. However, I began to notice that an unacceptable percentage of patients with various nerve related conditions either responded poorly to the treatments or not at all. A colleague who I shared office space with at the time employed acupuncture with his patients along with chiropractic. We had an agreement that entailed treating one another's patients when re-licensure training necessitated our traveling out of town. Upon return from a one of the seminars I attended, I noticed that several of my patients whom had otherwise not responded to my best efforts to resolved their health challenges got better while receiving a combination of acupressure/acupuncture and chiropractic care. I was surprised, and somewhat embarrassed but also very pleased with their dramatic improvements. After learning how the integration of acupressure/acupuncture helped my most difficult cases, I decided enroll in acupuncture training courses.

In the mid eighties, much scientific information began to come out about how various vitamins, minerals, herbs, amino acids and other natural remedies may help to prevent and/or ameliorate many health concerns. I decided to enroll in a three year Diplomat in Clinical Nutrition program. I completed the first half of the program while residing in Colorado.

After practicing in Colorado for over a decade my family and I moved to Phoenix, Arizona where I operated a busy practice for another decade. It was there that I continued training in clinical nutrition and subsequently became double board certified. While practicing in Arizona, I became interested in a new medical specialty called Anti-aging Medicine and eventually went on to receive board certification. My goal was to further help those patients who came to me with various nerve related conditions that either weren't responding or weren't completely resolved. These challenges included, but were not limited to, nerve pain, numbness, tingling, Carpal Tunnel Syndrome, Peripheral Neuropathy, Bell's Palsy, Sciatica, Shingles, Neuralgia, and symptoms of burning sensations and pins and needles. To my amazement, many of the difficult to resolve nerve conditions that previously had failed to fully respond and even those that didn't respond at all in the past, started to get better or completely resolve. Needless to say, my patients were elated and I was very humbled by their appreciation.

As my confidence in helping patients with challenging nerve disorders grew, I wanted to find a way to reach others who were in need of help. A colleague who hosted a weekend talk radio show on the subject of health invited me to be a guest on his program. I was asked to discuss how stress affects health in general, and the importance of having a healthy nervous system. Although this task seemed like more stress to my own nervous system than it was worth (having never appeared on a radio show before) I accepted the challenge. I enjoyed the experience so much that I decided to seek out a way to host my own health talk radio show.

I've been hosting my own talk radio show on health for 30+ years. This has required a lot of reading and research on my part in an effort to bring my radio audience and patients the latest breakthroughs in health, wellness, and lifestyle management. Over the years I have accumulated scientific evidence about how various nerve related challenges can be successfully helped through the use of non-pharmaceutical and non-surgical means. My clinical experience has taught me that many people with nerve disorders are often unnecessarily treated with pharmaceuticals that cause potent adverse side effects, and countless others have undergone dangerous, risky, and unnecessary surgeries to no avail.

Secret Nerve Cures was written in an effort to help those who suffer from nerve disorders. The information found in this book is not readily apparent in any other format. It is my hope that the information found within will help you discover a restoration to health, a remedy, or a method of treatment that you might not have considered before. It is my sincere desire through this book, Secret Nerve Cures, I will be able to share my knowledge and experiences in order to better serve and help educate others in finding safe, effective, cost effective, and science based treatments for nerve related challenges or concerns.

Some people have accused me of disseminating
objective, honest, and reliable health related information
—guilty as charged.

–Dr. Bob Martin

Chapter One
WHY WE HAVE
NERVES

The nervous system is an amazing thing.

It is responsible for sending, receiving, and processing information. It can sense your external and internal surroundings and then communicate this information between your brain, spinal cord, and other tissues in your body.

All of the organs, glands and muscles inside the body rely upon these nerve impulses. The information is used to coordinate voluntary movements such as talking, writing, or walking. Nerve impulses can help the body sense what is going on around it by touch, vision or other sensory means. The nervous system also controls our involuntary actions like breathing, digestion, blood pressure, body temperature, and the beating of our heart.

The best way to be healthy is to be informed.

Nerves are just one of the four types of tissues in the body:

Skin
Muscle
Connective tissue
Nerves

How do nerves work?

The nervous system is composed of the central nervous system and the peripheral nervous system. The brain is the center of the nervous system. Together, the brain and spinal cord form the central nervous system. Four other branches of nerves are considered the connections to the rest of the body. These connectors are often referred to as the peripheral nervous system.

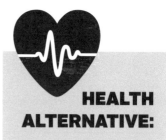

A nerve is like a cable that passes an electric current; it carries signals and vital information from one part of the body to another. The information is conveyed by using electrochemical impulses. These impulses happen almost instantaneously, allowing you to quickly move your hand from a hot surface, or dodge away from a flying object.

I'll be your designated driver on the highway to health.

The peripheral nervous system consists of more than 100 billion nerve cells that run throughout the body like strings, making connections with the brain, other parts of the body, and often with each other.

http://www.merck.com/mmhe/sec06/ch076/ch076d.html

Depending on their function, nerves are categorized into three groups —sensory nerves, autonomic nerves and motor nerves. Sensory nerves conduct sensory information to the central nervous system. Some type of sensory input, like vision, touch or sound activates these nerves. Autonomic nerves regulate body functions that cannot be controlled consciously, such as digestion, breathing, and heart functions. The

Your body didn't come with an owner's manual, so I'm here for you.

Sensory nerves: Sensory nerves help deliver information to the five senses: hearing, seeing, smelling, feeling, and tasting.

Autonomic nerves: affect internal organ functions like digestion or breathing.

Motor nerves: affect muscles and produce motion. They make something happen. Motor nerves control the movement of muscles responsible for walking, picking things up, or talking.

enteric nervous system is a division of the autonomic nervous system. It is the intrinsic nervous system of the gastrointestinal tract. The ENS has extensive connections with the central nervous system. It works in concert with the CNS to control the physiological demands of the body. Motor nerves conduct signals from the central nervous system back to the muscles. These nerves are responsible for movement, like moving the arm or the leg.

Why is nerve health so important?

Because nerves are crucial to almost everything we do, their health becomes vital to our health and wellbeing. Damage or interference to nerve function can occur by injury, swelling, infection, nutrient deficiency and/or lifestyle abuses. Sometimes damage can be caused from autoimmune diseases, diabetes, or failure of the blood vessels surrounding the nerve. This damage or malfunction is often manifest by pain, numbness, weakness, or even paralysis. Sometimes

HEALTH OUTRAGE:

Diseases of the nervous system afflict people of all ages throughout the world, inflict an enormous burden in lost life, disability, and suffering, and cost billions of dollars each year in medical expenses and reduced productivity.

(NINDS) 2011 http://www.istockphoto.com/file_thumbview_approve/6948492/2/istockphoto_6948492-grunge-set.jpg

a person will experience referred pain, which is when symptoms are felt in areas of the body that are far away from the actual site of damage. Damaged nerves may send messages too slowly or at the wrong times. Sometimes damaged nerves stop sending messages completely. Therefore, the health of our nerves becomes essential to the health of our body.

By the numbers

100 billion	The average human brain has about 100 billion nerve cells
170 mph	Nerve impulses to and from the brain travel as fast as 170 miles per hour
45 miles	There are 45 miles of nerves in the skin of a human being
1000	A nerve can send up to 1000 impulses per second
Nerves	The longest human nerve called; sciatic, is located in the leg and extends from the large toe to the spinal cord
12,000	One square inch of skin on the back of your hand has 12,000 nerve endings

The only bad health question is the one you're not asking. What does the autonomic nerve system look like inside my body?

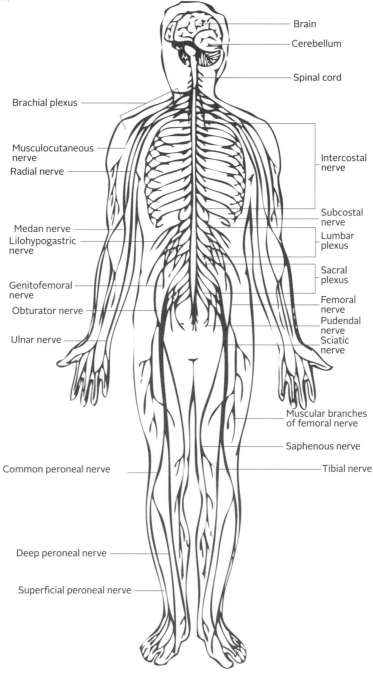

Brain

Cerebellum

Spinal cord

Brachial plexus

Musculocutaneous nerve

Radial nerve

Intercostal nerve

Subcostal nerve

Medan nerve

Lilohypogastric nerve

Lumbar plexus

Sacral plexus

Genitofemoral nerve

Obturator nerve

Femoral nerve

Pudendal nerve

Ulnar nerve

Sciatic nerve

Muscular branches of femoral nerve

Saphenous nerve

Common peroneal nerve

Tibial nerve

Deep peroneal nerve

Superficial peroneal nerve

Chapter Two
Nerve Challenges are
COMMON

Nerve pain or discomfort is often a symptom that accompanies several different conditions. In the beginning it is irritating and often frustrating. But as life goes on and symptoms don't improve it can become devastating, often bringing life changes that cause discouragement and even depression.

This ongoing pain can disrupt every aspect of life, both at work and at home. It places limits and sets boundaries on your decisions. Often nerve pain accompanies other life changing conditions such as diabetes or cancer. Adding the misery of nerve damage can make living with that condition even harder.

Your body didn't come with an owner's manual, so I'm here for you.

Symptoms of Nerve Damage:

Pain	Hypersensitive areas of the skin
Numbness	Hair loss on the affected part
Burning sensation	Shiny skin
Tingling	Weakness
Lancinating (shooting) pain	Muscle atrophy (loss of muscle tissue)
	(*JAMA vol. 299 No. 9, March 5, 2008*)

Many of these nerve related challenges can turn into unsolved or misunderstood health problems that remain undiagnosed or go without appropriate treatment for months or years. Sadly, this is a phenomenon that is common throughout the world.

How does nerve damage happen?

Nerve challenges are more common than you might think. This is because damage to nerves can happen in many different ways. Physical injury or trauma is the most common cause. Broken bones, car accidents, and sports injuries are other causes of nerve damage. Sometimes nerve damage can be caused by a disease. Both metabolic and endocrine disorders can affect nerves. In fact, Diabetes is a leading cause of peripheral neuropathy in the United States. Other health issues

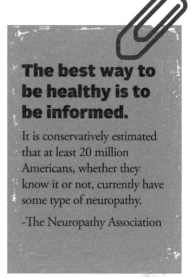

The best way to be healthy is to be informed.

It is conservatively estimated that at least 20 million Americans, whether they know it or not, currently have some type of neuropathy.

-The Neuropathy Association

that affect the nerves are hormonal imbalances, vitamin deficiencies, vascular damage, kidney disorders, chronic inflammation, spinal misalignment, cancers, and toxins —even repetitive stress can be a culprit. Infections and autoimmune disorders can also cause damage. Epstein-Barr virus, shingles, Lyme disease, HIV and herpes would be examples of viruses that can damage sensory nerves.

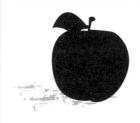

If you desire abundant health and wellness, you've come to the right place.

More than 100 types of peripheral neuropathy have been identified, each with its own characteristic set of symptoms, pattern of development, and prognosis.

NINDS/NIH

What happens when a nerve becomes damaged?

Nerve challenges often arise when there is damage to the nervous system. Nerve damage is anything that occurs to a nerve that alters its structure or function. Damaged nerves can interfere with the vital connections that relay information to and from the brain. Sometimes the messages are distorted, other times they might be interrupted. Because every nerve has a highly specific function within the body, its inability to communicate with the rest of the body soon becomes apparent. There are many different ways these failures manifest; the occurrences become classified as symptoms of someone who is experiencing nerve damage.

There is a wide array of symptoms that are experienced when nerves are damaged. You might experience tingling or pricking sensations. You may notice temporary numbness, sensitivity to touch, muscle weakness, or pain. These are all common symptoms. Sometimes people experience more extreme symptoms, which might include burning pain, stabbing sensation, paralysis, or muscle wasting. Some people even experience organ or gland dysfunction. The symptoms may appear suddenly, or they may be barely noticeable and progress slowly.

Damage affects each of the nerve groups differently.

Motor Nerve Damage is most often manifest through muscle weakness. Other symptoms include muscle twitching, painful cramps, bone degeneration and muscle loss. You may even notice changes in your skin, hair, and nails.

Sensory Nerve Damage is most often described by numbness in the hands and feet. It becomes harder to feel vibrations or adequately respond to touch. Sensory damage can also affect balance and cause neuropathic pain. If the smaller sensory fibers are damaged it might affect the body's ability to sense an injury or even an infection.

Autonomic Nerve Damage can become life threatening. If your breathing is affected, or if your heart begins to beat irregularly you may be experienc-

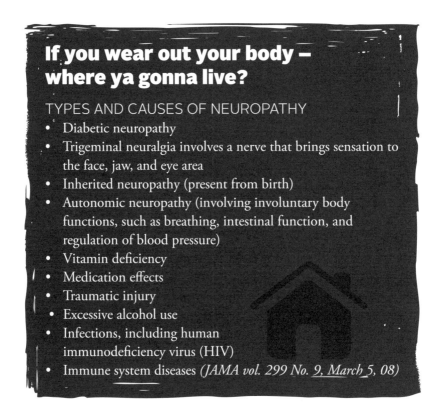

If you wear out your body – where ya gonna live?

TYPES AND CAUSES OF NEUROPATHY
- Diabetic neuropathy
- Trigeminal neuralgia involves a nerve that brings sensation to the face, jaw, and eye area
- Inherited neuropathy (present from birth)
- Autonomic neuropathy (involving involuntary body functions, such as breathing, intestinal function, and regulation of blood pressure)
- Vitamin deficiency
- Medication effects
- Traumatic injury
- Excessive alcohol use
- Infections, including human immunodeficiency virus (HIV)
- Immune system diseases *(JAMA vol. 299 No. 9, March 5, 08)*

ing a symptom that would require emergency medical care. Autonomic nerve damage can cause you to sweat abnormally or lose bladder control. It can affect the body's control over blood pressure, which could cause dizziness, lightheadedness and sometimes fainting.

The Good News Is...

Peripheral nerves, which connect our central nervous system to our limbs and organs, have an astonishing ability to regenerate after injury. With the help of fibroblasts, Schwann cells within the body can help repair the nerves. The fibroblasts send a signal to the Schwann cells, causing them to group together and guide the regrowth of axons across the wounded nerve. This new finding might lead to ways to improve the repair of peripheral nerves, and staying abreast of this research is important for those who suffer from damaged nerves.

Diagnosing Nerve Pain

A healthcare provider can help you determine if the pain you are suffering from is related to nerve dysfunction or damage. There are several tests that can be done including a neurological and orthope-

You've got health questions – I've got health answers. About 60 percent to 70 percent of people with diabetes have mild to severe forms of nervous system damage. Diabetic neuropathy is the most common type of neuropathy and affects up to two-thirds of patients with type 1 and type 2 diabetes. Diabetic neuropathy often involves the feet and legs and is responsible for lack of sensation, pain, poor coordination, burning sensation, pins and needles sensation etc.. ease of injury, infections and potential complications necessitating amputation. (*JAMA vol. 299 No. 9, March 5, 2008*

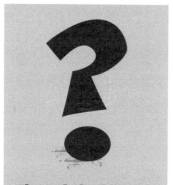

dic exam, a CT (computerized axial tomography) scan, nerve conduction studies, and MRI (magnetic resonance imaging.) In fact, there are even skin biopsies that can be done to examine the nerve endings.

Take the time to find the healthcare provider that is right for you and for your condition. A 1999 study reported in the Journal of Neurology stated that only 30% of neurologists surveyed believed they had been adequately trained to diagnose pain disorders, and only 20% thought they were properly trained to treat them. Some effort may be required to locate a provider that will be the best for your needs.

If you have an underlying disease such as cancer, diabetes, alcoholism, multiple sclerosis or another chronic condition, your healthcare provider can help you determine the best treatment for that disease. Sometimes improving the underlying condition can help slow the nerve damage or prevent it completely.

Nerve Damage Knows No Bounds

Nerve damage is prolific in our society today. Because there are so many risk factors the odds that someone will experience a nerve challenge sometime in their lifetime increase dramatically. Between genetics, toxins, viruses, immune disorders, chronic illnesses, and injuries, chances are high that at some point your nerves will be targeted. In fact, experts believe that between 2% - 8% of the general population live with nerve pain. The perception of nerve pain and/or discomfort may arise from multiple causes, and may be expressed subjectively by individuals in a multitude of ways. The damage knows no bounds, affecting men and women, adults and children from every walk of life and throughout the entire world. Therefore it becomes vitally important to understand how your nerves work, to learn to recognize the symptoms of damage, and to learn what you can do to maintain and restore your nerves to optimal health.

By the numbers How many people in the U.S. have nerve related challenges?

60-70%	Diabetic Neuropathy affects 60-70%
80%	Low Back Pain affects 80% of people at some point in their lifetime
8%	Musculoskeletal disorders, including Carpal Tunnel Syndrome affects 8%
5000	Bell's Palsy affects 1 of every 5000 people
1 million	Shingles affects 1 million American's a year
1.7 million	Trigeminal Neuralgia affects 1.7 million people in the US
80%	Neck Pain over 80% of adults are affected by neck pain.

Chapter Three
Nerves Under
SIEGE

Chances are you have already experienced some of the most common nerve challenges. Perhaps you are experiencing symptoms right now. Diseased or damaged nerves can cause neuropathy, sciatica, nerve pain, burning or tingling, carpal tunnel syndrome, facial pain or paralysis, numbness, and many other symptoms or conditions.

There are more than 100 different kinds of nerve disorders. Some nerve disorders can be genetically inherited. Others may occur over time, or come from injury or trauma, substance abuse, or exposure to toxins. Sometimes they are difficult to diagnose, and often they are hard to treat. In this chapter we will address some of the most common types of nerve disorders. Because every nerve has a specialized function, a wide array of symptoms can occur within the body as a result of each of these disorders. On the following pages each nerve disorder will be identified with its own set of symptoms, possible causes, and natural care options. For more options please refer to the chapters toward the end of the book, which will address possible remedies or treatment options in more detail.

Bell's Palsy:

Bell's palsy is a form of temporary facial paralysis. Symptoms usually begin suddenly and reach their peak within the first 48 hours. Bell's palsy affects about 23 out of 100,00 people at some time. It may result from injury, trauma, or from a herpes simplex viral infection. Most people begin to get better within two weeks and recover completely within three to six months. Healthcare providers will often tell people the condition may resolve in a matter of weeks, but unfortunately symptoms may last months or even take a year or more to completely resolve.

Standard medical care including the use of OTC (over-the-counter) drugs, prescription drugs or surgery – does little or nothing to help this mysterious and hard to manage condition. In fact, medical care may actually slow the healing process or make the condition worse. Conversely, safe, effective and inexpensive natural treatment remedies and modalities including specific vitamins, herbs, homeopathic remedies, and various forms of physical treatment such as chiropractic and acupuncture have proven effective.

Symptoms:

- Pain behind the ear
- Twitching
- Facial Weakness
- Facial Paralysis
- Face feels numb or heavy
- Drooling

- Drooping eyelid
- Dry eyes
- Eye pain
- Loss of taste
- Excessive tearing

Carpal Tunnel Syndrome:

Carpal Tunnel Syndrome may be caused by repetitive stress to the wrist joint, overt trauma, irritation and/or subsequent compression of a key nerve in the wrist. Women are three times as likely as men to develop carpal tunnel syndrome, and more than eight million people are affected by carpal tunnel syndrome each year. It is a painful and progressive condition. Symptoms usually start gradually and then worsen. Treatment involves resting the hand and wrist for at least two weeks. The majority of patients with Carpal Tunnel recover completely provided they receive proper treatment.

An optimal treatment regimen often includes rest, wrist bracing support, ice, and/or moist heat, chiropractic manipulation, acupuncture, ultrasound, and eventual physical rehabilitative exercise including reverse wrist curls using a form of resistance. Supplementing with specific vitamins, minerals, herbs and homeopathic remedies can be very important. Additionally, the use of topical botanicals, and homeopathic analgesic formulation are often helpful.

Other common peripheral nerve injuries include

Cubital tunnel syndrome, which is caused by increased pressure to the ulnar nerve, the nerve just next to the interior elbow. Radial tunnel syndrome, which affects the nerve that originates at the neck and travels along the back of the arm to the hand.

Symptoms:

- Tingling or numbness in fingers or hand
- Pain radiating from wrist to shoulder
- Pain radiates down into palm or fingers
- A sense of weakness in the hand
- A tendency to drop objects

Diabetic Neuropathy:

Diabetic Neuropathy is a peripheral nerve disorder. This disorder is caused by poor blood sugar control. The most common type of diabetic neuropathy is usually manifest in the feet, but may also progress upward to include legs, arms and hands. Most often it develops slowly, but it may occur early in the disease. Controlling blood sugar levels can prevent tissue damage. Treating or properly managing diabetes my stop the progression and improve symptoms. Recovery is slow. However, this condition responds well to many of the natural treatments and modalities described in this book. Additionally, vitamin, botanical and homeopathic remedies are helpful.

Symptoms:
- Numbness, tingling in the feet or lower legs
- Intense pain
- Loss of sensation in the feet
- Difficulty walking
- Weakness in the foot muscles
- Burning Sensation
- Increased Sensitivity

Paresthesia:

Paresthesia is a condition in which a person feels numbness, tingling, prickling or a sensation of burning. This sensation most often occurs in the extremities. Paresthesia is often a symptom of another disease, disorder, or condition. It can result from inflammation, infection, trauma or malignancy. Sometimes paresthesia sensations are short-term and disappear quickly. Paresthesia can also be chronic. It generally indicates that there is damage or some type of interference to the nerves. Many types of paresthesias originate as a result of spinal misalignments in the neck or back regions called subluxations. The doctor of choice in non-fracture related paresthesias is a Doctor of Chiropractic (see Chapter Eleven). Additionally, vitamin, botanical and homeopathic remedies are helpful.

Symptoms:
• Burning
• Tingling
• Numbness
• Prickling
• Skin crawling
• Itching
• Pins and needles
• Most often occurs in the arms, legs, hands, feet or face.

Skin Sensory Nerves:

Nerve endings in the skin can cause chronic pain in conditions such as diabetes or shingles. Problems with nerve endings may contribute to painful conditions such as fibromyalgia, or migraine headaches. Damage to these nerves may also contribute to symptoms associated with shingles, complex regional pain syndrome (formerly called Reflex Sympathetic Dystrophy,) carpal tunnel syndrome, psoriasis, sciatica, and other neurological problems. Chronic numbness, pain and itching sensations can also manifest from chemotherapy and unintended side effects caused by many over-the-counter and/or prescription drugs.

Symptoms:
- Pain
- Itching
- Tingling
- Numbness
- Burning Sensation
- Pins and needles
- Stabbing Pain

Autonomic Nerve Damage:

Autonomic nerve damage affects the involuntary or partially voluntary activities of your body. This damage may affect your heart, blood pressure, and digestion. Causes may include alcoholism, autoimmune diseases, tumors, traumatic injury, spinal misalignment, nutritional deficiencies and chronic illness. Vitamin, botanical and homeopathic remedies are helpful.

Symptoms:
- Too much sweating
- Inability to sense chest pain
- Lightheadedness
- Dry eyes and mouth
- Constipation
- Bladder dysfunction
- Sexual dysfunction

Motor Nerve Damage:

Motor nerve damage affects your movement and actions. This type of nerve damage affects essential muscle activity such as speaking, walking, breathing and swallowing. Cancers, toxic drugs, trauma, spinal misalignment, or environmental toxins can trigger damage. Environmental and genetic factors may also play a role. Additionally, vitamin, botanical and homeopathic remedies are helpful.

Symptoms:
• Weakness
• Muscle atrophy
• Twitching
• Paralysis

Sensory Nerve Damage:

Sensory nerve damage affects your ability to relay information from your skin and muscles to your spinal cord and brain. Damage to these fibers lessens the ability to feel vibrations and touch. Balance can also be affected by damaged sensory nerves. Additionally, vitamin, botanical and homeopathic remedies are helpful.

Symptoms:
• Pain
• Sensitivity
• Numbness
• Tingling or prickling
• Burning
• Loss of balance

Brain Damage:

Brain damage or brain injury is defined as the destruction or degeneration of brain cells. Brain damage may occur due to a wide range of conditions, illnesses, or injuries.

Possible causes of brain damage include, a dysfunctional hereditary gene, oxygen deprivation, poisoning, infection, tumor formation, physical trauma and degenerative neurological illness

The brain is the most complex organ in the human body, and perhaps the most remarkable. Scientists believe the brain is often capable of self repair depending on the extent to which injury has occurred.

There are many effective ways to help individuals challenged by brain damage, and they include; physical therapy, exercise rehabilitation, occupational therapy, speech and language therapy and psychological support.

Whether a person is attempting to prevent, mitigate, or rehabilitate with respect to brain health in-general - conservative, safe and effective treatment(s) exist today. Protocols to consider include; HBOT (hyperbaric oxygen therapy), vitamin therapy, botanicals and amino acids.

University of Wisconsin – Milwaukee, and Nobel Prize winning research recently lead to the discovery of a special calcium binding protein found only in jellyfish called; aequorin. The reason this unique protein discovery is important has to do with its ability to bind calcium in the human brain. Excess calcium is thought to cause inflammation within brain neurons leading to potential damage. As we age into our 40's and beyond and start to experience memory lapses such as misplacing or forgetting where we put our car keys, not being able to remember people's names, walking into a room and forgetting what we intended to do and so on may indicate that excess or unbound brain calcium is negatively impacting our ability to have healthy brain function, clear thinking and optimal memory. These unfortunate events associated with the aging process are thought to contribute to an increase risk or Alzheimer's, Parkinson's and other degenerative brain diseases.

Several years ago, a Wisconsin based nutraceutical company by the name of Quincy Bioscience discovered a way to develop a protein binding compound identical that which occurs naturally in jellyfish. This supplement, Prevagen, is available in most food stores.

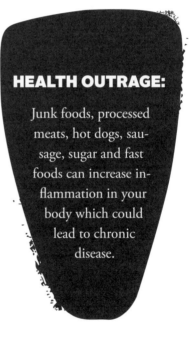

HEALTH OUTRAGE:

Junk foods, processed meats, hot dogs, sausage, sugar and fast foods can increase inflammation in your body which could lead to chronic disease.

Symptoms:

- Cognitive
- Perceptual
- Physical
- Behavioral
- Emotional

Nerve Pain:

Nerve Pain may have no obvious cause. Sometimes it can be caused by spinal misalignment to Multiple sclerosis, shingles, or diabetes. Alcoholism can also cause nerve pain. Surgery, amputation, infections, medical drugs including chemotherapy, or other nerve pain can be a chronic pain state in which the nerve fibers may be damaged, dysfunctional or injured.

Symptoms:
• Shooting pain
• Burning pain
• Tingling
• Numbness
• Dull Pain
• Throbbing Pain

Cramps

Cramps are a painful, involuntary and often spasmodic contraction of the muscles. The uncontrolled contraction happens unexpectedly. Cramps may affect any muscle, but are most common in the legs, feet, and hands. They are a common symptom of nerve and neurological challenges. Metabolic and nutrient deficiencies may also play a role.

Symptoms:
• Intense localized muscle pain
• Pain is often debilitating
• Pain comes on quickly and fades gradually
• Muscle spasms

Neuralgia:

Neuralgia is nerve pain that is severe. There are two types of neuralgia. Trigeminal neuralgia is severe facial nerve pain resulting from the swelling of the trigeminal nerve. Postherpetic neuralgia is nerve pain that is constant and severe and sometimes occurs as a result of shingles. Most neuralgias respond to conservative non-drug treatments and remedies. Additionally, vitamin, botanical and homeopathic remedies are helpful.

Symptoms of Trigeminal neuralgia include:

• A severe stabbing pain in your face.
• Pain is usually felt in the jaw, cheek, eye or forehead
• Pain is generally on one side of face
• Tingling or numbness may be present just before pain
• Burning may occur just after the attack

Postherpetic Neuralgia symptoms include:

• Constant burning or throbbing pain
• Occasional stabbing or shooting pain
• Intense itching

Occipital Neuralgia:

A term used to describe a cycle of pain originating from the suboccipital area (base of the skull.) Pain often radiates to the back front and side of the head, as well as behind the eyes and can be caused by spinal injury such as whiplash or compression of nerves in the spinal column.

Symptoms

• Headache
• Stiff neck
• Muscle soreness or spasm
• Pain behind eyes

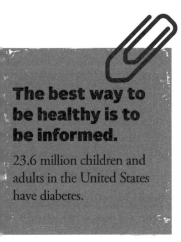

Sciatica:

Sciatica is a low back pain most often described as a deep, severe pain that shoots down the buttock and the leg. It is usually worse after prolonged sitting and standing. The sciatic nerves are the largest nerves in the body and go from the low back, behind the hip joint, down the buttock and then down the back of the leg to the foot. The pain is often described as a shooting pain.

Symptoms:
• Pain running from low back down thigh and calf
• Numbness or muscle weakness in leg or foot
• Tingling or pins-and-needles

Tarsal Tunnel Syndrome

The tarsal tunnel, also known as posterior tibial neuralgia, is in the foot between bones and overlying fibrous tissue on the inside of the heel. Tarsal tunnel syndrome is when this nerve is pinched and can be very painful. This condition is very similar to carpal tunnel syndrome except happens in the foot or heel region.

Symptoms:
• Pain
• Parasthesias
• Numbness
• Foot muscle atrophy

Shingles:

Shingles is a virus that causes a rash or blisters on the skin. It is related to chickenpox. The first sign of shingles is often a tingling pain. After several days a rash of blisters appears. Shingle pain can be mild or intense. Some people experience itching, others feel pain from even a gentle touch. The most common place for shingles to appear is around the trunk or waistline. For most people the symptoms subside within three to five weeks.

Symptoms:
- Headache
- Sensitivity to light
- Flu-like symptoms
- Itching
- Tingling
- Band of pain
- Rash with blisters

A conservative approach for relief may include:
- Black elderberry extract
- Olive leaf extract
- Echinacea
- Wakanaga Kyolic- Aged Garlic Extract
- Vitamins A, B, C and E
- Topical cream or lotion containing Capsaicin
- Calamine Lotion can also be helpful

If you wear out your body – where ya gonna live?

10 % of people who have had chicken pox as children will get shingles as adults.

Peripheral Neuropathy:

Peripheral Neuropathy is a lack of sensation in the extremities. It is usually symmetrical from the spine down to the extremities. This type of neuropathy usually begins in the toes and continues upwards. If the pattern continues up the calf, hands and fingertips may become affected over time. True peripheral neuropathy eventually involves all of the extremities including both hands and both feet. Many medical medications or drugs can also cause a peripheral neuropathy. Vitamin, botanical and homeopathic remedies are helpful.

Symptoms:
- Numbness and tingling that begins in feet and hands and spreads to legs and arms.
- Burning pain
- Extreme sensitivity to touch
- Jabbing pain
- Extreme sensitivity to touch
- Lack of coordination
- Muscle weakness
- Bowel or bladder problems

Small Fiber Neuropathy:

Small Fiber Neuropathy results from damage to the nerve fibers that convey pain and temperature sensations. The small fiber nerves are found near the surface of our skin. They allow us to feel heat or cold. Damage to these nerves will sometimes cause loss of sensation; other times it causes extreme sensitivity. Because of this, symptoms can include pain and hypersensitivity, but they can also include a lack of sensitivity to pain. Clothes can feel like sandpaper, hands may become overly sensitive to touch and, pressure from shoes can cause severe pain in the feet. However, sometimes the loss of these small fibers may also cause an inability to feel pain. In these situations, some people will sustain wounds or injuries without even noticing. Small Fiber Neuropathy is usually localized to the feet, arms and hands and is a condition that is often undiagnosed or misdiagnosed.

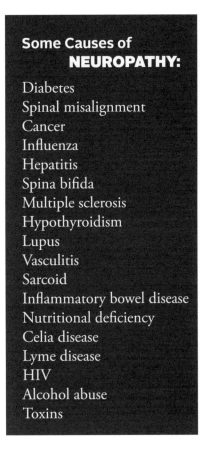

Some Causes of NEUROPATHY:

Diabetes
Spinal misalignment
Cancer
Influenza
Hepatitis
Spina bifida
Multiple sclerosis
Hypothyroidism
Lupus
Vasculitis
Sarcoid
Inflammatory bowel disease
Nutritional deficiency
Celia disease
Lyme disease
HIV
Alcohol abuse
Toxins

Symptoms:

- Severe pain
- Diminished thermal perception
- Diminished pain perception
- Burning pain
- Prickling pain
- Stabbing pain
- Jabbing pain

The Condition You're In Determines the Condition You're In

Sometimes nerve damage comes as a complication from another disease. Nerve damage is often a symptom of another condition. For example, approximately 70% of people with diabetes will develop Peripheral Neuropathy. Cancer patients who receive chemotherapy or radiation may also develop nerve related damage and experience symptoms. Some common conditions that lead to or may be associated with nerve disorders are listed below.

Complex Regional Pain Syndrome

Complex Regional Pain Syndrome (CRPS) (formerly known as Reflex Sympathic Dystrophy) is an unusual chronic pain condition that mainly affects the arms and legs. CRPS is most likely to occur due as a result of trauma to an extremity that requires immobilization, such as fracture, surgery, or severe trauma, like a gunshot wound. However, lesser injuries such as neck and back sprains or even the act of drawing blood may generate this condition in some individuals.

Symptoms:
- Extreme skin sensitivity
- Intense burning pain
- Muscle contractions
- Joint stiffness
- Muscle atrophy

Some causes of CRPS
- Trauma requiring immobilization
- Fracture
- Surgery
- Gun shot wounds
- Sprains
- Blood draw

Diabetes:

There are two types of diabetes. Juvenile or Type 1 diabetes is usually diagnosed in children and young adults. In type 1 diabetes, the pancreas no long produces insulin. Type 2 diabetes is the most common form of diabetes. Millions of Americans have been diagnosed with Type 2 diabetes, and many more live without knowing that they are at high risk. In type 2 diabetes your body is resistant to the effects of insulin — a hormone that regulates the movement of sugar into your cells — or your body doesn't produce enough insulin to maintain a normal glucose level. Without the proper use of insulin in the body high blood glucose levels occur, causing damage to the body. Prolonged exposure to high blood glucose levels is thought to be the root cause of nerve damage. All types of nerves can be impacted from poor glucose control. Vitamin, botanical and homeopathic remedies are helpful.

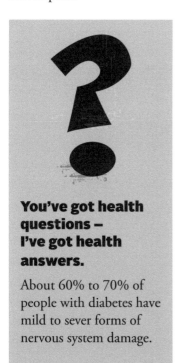

You've got health questions – I've got health answers.

About 60% to 70% of people with diabetes have mild to sever forms of nervous system damage.

Symptoms:
- Frequent urination
- Unusual thirst
- Extreme hunger
- Fatigue
- Irritability
- Blurred vision
- Frequent infections
- Weight loss or gain
- Slow wound healing

Fibromyalgia:

Fibromyalgia is a common arthritis-related illness and can often be misdiagnosed and misunderstood. It is often characterized by chronic widespread pain. It is estimated to affect two to four percent of the population. Research indicates that often abnormalities within the central nervous system may be linked to the clinical symptoms associated with Fibromyalgia. The symptoms of Fibromyalgia are often magnified by malfunctions in the way the nervous system processes pain. Possible causes could include: unresolved infections, nutritional deficiencies, sleep dysfunctions, endocrine imbalances leading to hormone disturbance, unhealthy lifestyle, lack of spinal hygiene (chiropractic care). Also, consider a Comprehensive Digestive Test (CDT) and Comprehensive Nutrition Analysis (CNBA) (See companies I recommend: Nutritional Testing Services at back of book.)

Symptoms:
- Dizziness
- Numbness or tingling in the face, arms, hands, legs, or feet
- Moderate or severe fatigue
- Decreased energy
- Chronic muscle pain
- Muscle spasms or tightness
- Weakness in the limbs
- Difficulty concentrating
- Abdominal pain, bloating, nausea
- Migraine headaches
- Jaw and facial tenderness

Multiple Sclerosis:

Multiple Sclerosis is a disease that affects the brain and spinal cord. It is an autoimmune disease that results in loss of muscle control, balance, vision, and sensations. Common early symptoms include numbness, pins and needles sensations, in coordination, weakness especially in the legs, painful loss of vision in one eye, double vision, dizziness, pain at various sites, urinary symptoms and impotence. With Multiple Sclerosis one's own immune system damages the nerves of the brain and the spinal cord. Those with MS should consider reading a book entitled: *Dr. Swanks MS Diet.*

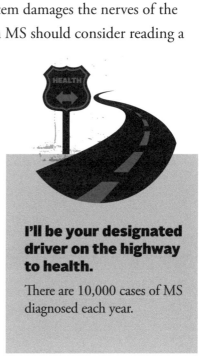

Symptoms:
- Tingling
- Numbness
- Loss of balance
- Weakness in one or more limbs
- Blurred vision
- Sensitivity to heat
- Fatigue

I'll be your designated driver on the highway to health.

There are 10,000 cases of MS diagnosed each year.

Lupus:

Lupus is a chronic inflammatory disease. It occurs when the body's immune system attacks its own organs and tissues. Most people with lupus will have episodes, or flare-ups, when symptoms get worse far a time and then improve or disappear for a while. Lupus can affect the nervous system and the brain. Peripheral neuropathy occurs in about 15% of patients with Lupus. For many Lupus patients nervous system involvement is completely reversible. A DHEA (dehydroepiandrosterone) blood test should be included in a Comprehensive Nutritional Blood Test/Analysis. Also, a DHEA value can be derived via salivary hormone testing (see page 175).

Symptoms:
- Fatigue
- Fever
- Joint pain
- Butterfly rash on the face
- Skin lesions that worsen with sun exposure
- Mouth sores
- Hair loss
- Easy bruising

This is a place where like-minded people gather to get well.

Approximately 1,500,000 Americans have been diagnosed with a form of Lupus.

Celiac Disease:

Celiac disease is an autoimmune disease where the immune system attacks gluten or gliadin and harms your small intestine. Gluten is a protein found in wheat, barley, oats, couscous, durum, kamut, semolina, spelt, triticale, and rye. Symptoms can come from both malabsorption and malnutrition including vitamin and mineral deficiencies. Deficiencies of B12 and thiamine may contribute to nerve damage. Low levels of potassium and magnesium can lead to severe muscle weakness and muscle cramps.

A recent study found that almost 10 percent of people with celiac disease suffer from peripheral neuropathy or ataxia. Some people with celiac disease suffer from neuropathic symptoms before they notice any gastrointestinal symptoms. Someone who suffers from neuropathy of an unknown cause should consider being tested for celiac disease. The most non-invasive way to test for Gluten Intolerance is through salivary testing. Blood tests and intestinal biopsies may also be used. A Salivary Hormone test should also be considered. (See Nutritional Testing Services on page 174). Those with celiac should consider adding grains such as brown rice, corn, millet, quinoa, and amaranth to their diet. A Comprehensive Digestive Analysis extended panel should also be considered. Consider a Comprehensive Digestive Test (CDT) in order to measure for a positive Gliadin antibody response (see page 171-173).

Symptoms:
- Gas and bloating
- Abdominal cramps
- Weight loss
- Feeling very tired
- Weakness
- Muscle Cramps
- Anemia
- Neuropathic symptoms
- Numbness, tingling or reduced sensation in the face and body

Epstein Barr:

An infection from the Epstein-Barr virus is very common. Nearly 95% of adults have had an Epstein-Barr infection. Usually the symptoms are mild, similar to a cold. Sometimes a more severe infection occurs. This is called infectious mononucleosis. Viruses like Epstein Barr and bacteria can attack nerve tissues and damage sensory nerves, causing pain. Consider a Comprehensive Digestive Test (CDT) and Comprehensive Nutritional Blood Analysis (CNBA) (See page 171-172 and 174).

Symptoms:
- Extreme fatigue
- Fever
- Sore throat
- Swollen lymph nodes
- Enlarged spleen

Your body didn't come with an owner's manual, so I'm here for you.

1 out of every 133 Americans has celiac disease

Restless Legs Syndrome:

Restless legs syndrome is characterized by an irresistible urge to move the legs, and is commonly experienced during times of rest. It is a neurological condition that can begin at any age and generally becomes worse as you get older. Restless legs syndrome can disrupt sleep. It affects up to ten percent of the population. For those suffering from RLS, it may be helpful to eliminate alcohol, caffeine, refined sugars, and tobacco. Increasing exercise may also help the condition. Many have tried calcium, magnesium, vitamin E and potassium prior to bedtime. Chiropractic, acupuncture, massage and herbal formulas should also be considered. Iron deficiency is a possible cause. Toxic metal and mineral analysis should be considered along with nutritional blood analysis. Consider a Comprehensive Nutritional Blood Analysis (CNBA) (See page 174).

Symptoms:
- Itching, tingling or crawling sensations within the legs and sometimes arms.
- Restlessness
- An urge to move the limbs
- Symptoms occur only while lying or sitting.
- Symptoms often improve with activity

Spinal Stenosis:

Spinal stenosis can cause pain or numbness. It occurs from a narrowing of one or more areas in your spine. Most often it occurs in the neck or lower back. The narrowing puts pressure on the spinal cord.

It is commonly caused by age-related changes, past trauma, or lack of spinal hygiene (chiropractic care). Standard care should be considered including anti-gravity inversion therepy, yoga, DRX-9000 (specialized form of spinal traction), low impact exercise and swimming.

Symptoms:
- Numbness
- Weakness
- Tingling
- Neck pain
- Shoulder pain
- Loss of bowel or bladder control
- Cramping in the legs

Hormonal Imbalance:

Hormonal Imbalance is caused when there is an incorrect relationship between progesterone, estrogen, testosterone, DHEA, thyroid hormone and others levels in the body. Variations in balance can have a dramatic effect on health. The hormones can vary depending on factors such as age, stress, nutrition, exercise, exposure to environmental toxins, ovulation and general lifestyle. Hormone imbalances can disturb normal metabolic processes thus causing neuropathies. Fluid retention and swollen tissues can exert pressure on peripheral nerves. A salivary hormone test panel and analysis should be considered (See page 175).

Symptoms:
- Depression, fatigue and anxiety
- Fibrocystic breasts
- Hair loss
- Facial hair growth
- Headaches
- Dizziness and foggy thinking
- Urinary tract infections

Inflammation:

Inflammation is sometimes caused when the immune system inappropriately triggers an inflammatory response when there are no foreign substances to fight off. Inflammation causes chemicals to be released into the affected tissues. Some of these chemicals can cause swelling to occur. The inflammatory process can also stimulate nerves and cause pain. Inflammation can cause neuritis, which affects the peripheral nerves, blocking sensory and motor functions. Consider a C-reactive protein blood test (See page 177).

Symptoms:
• Swollen joints or joint pain
• Joint stiffness
• Redness
• Fever
• Chills
• Fatigue
• Headaches
• Loss of appetite
• Muscle stiffness
• General pain
• Numbness
• Tingling
• Burning Sensation
• Pins and needles

Lyme Disease:

Lyme disease is an illness carried by ticks. An infected tick can transmit the illness to humans. Untreated, the bacteria will establish itself in various body tissues. Lyme disease can cause a number of symptoms, some of which are severe. If left untreated, infection can spread to the heart, joints, and the nervous system. Lyme disease is often treated with antibiotics and other integrative modalities. A specialized lyme disease blood test should be considered.

Symptoms:
- Rash
- Flu-like symptoms
- Migratory joint pain
- Neurological problems
- Numbness or weakness of limbs
- Impaired muscle movement
- Memory loss
- Difficulty concentrating

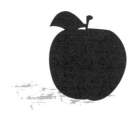

If you desire abundant health and wellness, you've come to the right place.

Tips to reduce your risk for Lyme disease

1. When outdoors in an area where ticks may be present, wear long sleeves and long pants tucked into socks.

2. After outdoor activities check for ticks, especially behind the knees, between fingers and toes, under the arms, and on top of the head.

3. Remove attached ticks promptly. Use tweezers, and grab the tic as close to the skin as possible.

Human immunodeficiency virus (HIV):

Human immunodefieciency virus is a virus that can cause acquired immunodeficiency syndrome (AIDS). This is a life-threatening condition in which the immune system begins to fail. HIV interferes with the body's ability to fight off disease and can also make the body more susceptible to infections the body would normally resist. HIV can cause extensive damage to the nervous system. Painful polyneuropathy of the hands and feet is often one of the first clinically apparent signs of HIV infection.

Symptoms:
• Lack of energy
• Weight loss
• Frequent fevers and sweats
• Persistent or frequent yeast infections
• Persistent skin rashes or flaky skin
• Short-term memory loss
• Mouth, genital or anal sores from herpes infections cough and shortness of breath
• Cough and shortness of breath
• Seizures
• Lack of coordination
• Difficult or painful swallowing
• Diarrhea
• Fever
• Vision loss
• Nausea
• Severe headaches

Toxins:

People who are exposed on a regular basis to lead, mercury, arsenic, solvents, pesticides, herbacides or other industrial drugs frequently develop neuropathy. Other environmental toxins can also cause peripheral nerve damage. Alcohol and many other medical drugs can damage nerves. These include nitrous oxide, colchicine, metronidazole, lithium, phenytoin, cimetidine, disulfiram, chloroquine, amitriptyline, thalidomide, cisplatin, paclitaxel.and many others. Consider a Toxic Metal and Mineral Test (See page 173-174).

Symptoms:
• Headaches
• Nausea
• Lung irritation
• Coughing
• Back pain
• Dizziness
• Depression
• Fatigue
• Rashes
• Infertility

Chapter Four
Nerve TOXINS

A toxin is a poisonous substance that is capable of causing disease. Neurotoxins are chemicals that injure cells in the nervous system. Some neurotoxins are mercury, alcohol, tobacco smoke and pesticides. Some chemicals can either slow the networking of neurons or completely prevent communication, which can impair the normal function of the brain and nervous system.

Unfortunately many of the foods available for purchase in a supermarket contain harmful ingredients. Labels are filled with ingredients such as refined sugar, artificial sweeteners, (aspartame, nutra sweet) MSG (monosodium glutamate), preservatives, harmful oils and food colorings, which can all have a negative effect on health, and may adversely impact nerve tissue.

In this chapter we will focus on some of the most common toxins and the effect they have on nerve health.

The best way to be healthy is to be informed.

Foods, drugs and other substances that can be toxic to the health of your nerve and overall health in general:
- Margarine, hydrogenated fats or partially hydrogenated fats
- Salt
- Chlorine
- Antibiotics
- Aspartame
- Mono Sodium Glutamate
- Pesticides
- Carcinogens
- Hormones
- Food additives
- Sugar
- Refined oils
- Junk foods/processed foods
- Fried foods
- Soft drinks
- Chemotherapy
- Mercury poisoning

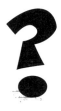

You've got health questions – I've got health answers.

Almost 50,000 cases of alcohol poisoning are reported each year.

Alcohol is a substance that can have a toxic effect on nerve tissue. Beer, wine and other liquors contain alcohol. Alcohol consumption can have a negative effect on your health. It is considered neurotoxic, which means it can directly destroys the nerve cells located in the central nervous system and the peripheral nervous system. The toxic effects alcohol has on nerve and muscles cells can be profound and may include poor coordination, sensory deficits, and weakness. Alcohol may also contribute to the development of neuropathy.

HEALTH OUTRAGE:

Alcohol abuse and Alcoholism are the third leading cause of preventable deaths in the US.

Lead is toxic to many organs and tissues in the body including the nervous system. In fact, lead is known to interfere with the development of the nervous system and is capable of interfering with a variety of the body processes. Primary sources of lead exposure are deteriorating lead-based paint and dust and soil that have been contaminated by lead. Water pipes, vinyl mini-blinds, fishing sinkers, leaded gasoline, costume jewelry and playground equipment can all contain lead. Consider a Toxic Metal and Mineral Test (See page 173-174).

Tobacco smoke contains toxins such as carbon monoxide and cyanide. The smoke can harm almost every organ of the body. Among other diseases, tobacco can cause cancer, heart disease, and respiratory diseases. Tobacco smoke has a toxic effect on health. The Centers for Disease Control and Prevention describes tobacco use as "the single most important preventable risk to human health." Smokers are twice as likely to develop neuropathy. Tobacco is a major cause of optic neuropathy and macular degeneration.

Your body didn't come with an owner's manual, so I'm here for you.

What is the first thing the US Surgeon General advises you to do to quit smoking?

Set a quit date. Schedule a visit to your health care provider before that date to get practical advice on a plan that will work best for you.

Mercury comes from industries and power plants and is released into our air, land and water. Sometimes toxic exposure happens when an item containing mercury breaks, such as a thermometer, dental filling, fluorescent light tube or an alkaline battery. Mercury is known to be a potent nerve toxin, and is capable of destroying the structure of the nerve. Avoid fish known to contain high levels of mercury such as, tilefish, shark, swordfish, king mackerel, tuna, and trout. For lead and metal poisioning, toxic metal and mineral analysis is recommended (See page 173-174).

Pesticides are toxic substances used to kill or control insects, weeds, rodents, bacteria and mildew. Some of these herbicides, insecticides and fungicides are harmful to humans. Chronic effects of exposure to certain pesticides can include nerve disorders. Insecticides generally cause the greatest number of pesticide poisonings because they inhibit the enzyme cholinesterase, which causes a disruption of the nervous system.

Organic solvents are commonly used in dry cleaning, nail polish removers, paint thinners, glue solvents, spot removers, detergents and perfumes. Toxic amounts of organic solvents have been shown to impair body balance, manual coordination and reaction times. Inhalation can produce symptoms that include drowsiness, headache, dizziness and nausea. Research shows that acute exposure in humans can include central nervous system depression and psychomotor impairment. Organic solvent exposure can also decrease motor and sensory nerve conduction. Organic acids urine test is recommended.

Carbon Monoxide gas is poisonous, and even a small amount can cause loss of consciousness and death. Carbon monoxide becomes dangerous once you have breathed it in. Inside your body it mixes with hemoglobin, which makes it so the blood can no longer carry oxygen. This mixing produces a compound called carboxyhemoglobin. This leads to swelling in the brain, which can cause unconsciousness, neurological damage, and death.

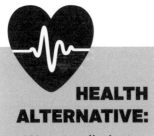

Artificial Sweeteners can have a toxic effect on nerve health. Aspartame, aka Equal and Nutrasweet, is an artificial sweetener commonly found in sugar free and diet products. Exposure to aspartame may cause headaches, dizziness, poor balance, memory loss, fatigue and other neurological symptoms. Some studies have shown that aspartame may aggravate or worsen several chronic neurological illnesses. Suggested reading includes, Excitotoxins: The Taste That Kills by Russell Blaylock, MD. Other artificial sweeteners to avoid include Acesulfame-K, aka acesulfame potassium, Sunette, Sweet One, Sweet 'n Safe, Saccharin, aka Sweet 'N Low, Sugar Twin, and Sucralose, aka Splenda.

Refined sugar is a sugar that has been depleted of its life forces, vitamins and minerals. Nutritionists suggest that refined sugar provides empty calories, lacking the natural minerals found in the sugar beet or sugar cane. The World Health Organization suggests that people should limit their daily consumption of sugar to less than 10 percent of their total energy intake. However, most people eat about 23 teaspoons of added sugar every

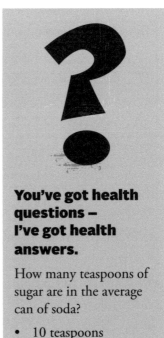

You've got health questions — I've got health answers.

How many teaspoons of sugar are in the average can of soda?

- 10 teaspoons

day. Sugar has been linked to kidney disease, diabetes, eye problems and severe nerve damage to the lower limbs and other parts of the body. Suggested reading includes Lick the Sugar Habit, and Suicide by Sugar by Nancy Appleton, PhD.

Safe/non toxic sweeteners include Stevia, Lo Han, Agave, and Xylitol. More information on Xylitol can be found at Xlear Corporation (www.xlear.com).

Monosodium glutamate (MSG) is a flavor enhancer that is commonly used in processed and prepackaged foods. MSG is considered an excitatory neurotransmitter, which means it can excite brain neurons and increase the levels of electrical activity in the brain. MSG breaks down into glutamate, which is an excitatory neuro-transmitter. Too much glutamate can activate the neurons into a continual firing mode causing them to eventually die. Because there is so much concern about MSG, the FDA commissioned a study to be conducted by the Federation of American Societies for Experimental Biology (FASEB). The study resulted in a 350-page report completed on July 31, 1995. The research determined that MSG consumption can result in the following side-effects:

- A burning sensation in the back of the neck, forearms and chest
- A numbness in the back of the neck, radiating to the arms and back
- Tingling,
- Warmth and weakness in the face, temples, upper back, neck and arms
- Facial pressure or tightness

- Chest pain
- Headache
- Nausea
- Rapid heartbeat
- Bronchospasm (difficulty breathing) in MSG-intolerant people with asthma
- Drowsiness
- Weakness

The following list gives some examples of how MSG is disguised, so that unsuspecting consumers aren't always aware that they're ingesting a potential nerve damaging substance. Also included below are foods and additives that often contain MSG or excitotoxins.

- Monosodium Glutamate
- Hydrolyzed Vegetable Protein
- Hydrolyzed Protein
- Hydrolyzed Plant Protein
- Plant Protein Extract
- Sodium Caseinate
- Calcium Caseinate
- Yeast Extract
- Textured Protein (Including TVP)
- Autolyzed Yeast
- Hydrolyzed Oat Flour
- Corn Oil
- Malt Extract
- Malt Flavoring
- Bouillon
- Broth
- Stock
- Flavoring
- Natural Flavors/Flavoring
- Seasoning
- Spices
- Carrageenan
- Enzymes
- Soy Protein Concentrate
- Soy Protein Isolate
- Whey Protein Concentrate

Sometimes glutamate is referred to as an excitotoxin. Suggested reading includes; *Monosodium Glutamate Danger* by John Erb, and *In Bad Taste* by George R. Schwartz

Some Effects from Exposure to Neurotoxins can include:

Aggressiveness

Compromised physical growth

Hyperactivity, poor attention span, or impulsiveness

Learning difficulty

Memory impairment

Mental retardation

Nerve damage

Poor motor coordination

Sensory processing problems

Speech difficulty

Social immaturity

Vision and hearing problems

Replace something you already do with something better:

_____

_____

_____

Chapter Five

Medical Drugs are Risky
BUSINESS

We live in a society filled with medical experts and drug giants. Research has led to the discovery of pharmaceutical drugs that provide disease management, but not necessarily a cure. While these drugs have been credited with saving thousands of lives every year and relieving much suffering, it is important to remain aware of the potential adverse side effects and negative influence they may have on your health. It is critically important for a patient to remain educated about the potential short and long-term harm that can come from taking over-the-counter and prescription drugs.

Often anticonvulsants or antidepressants will be prescribed to help combat and control nerve pain and discomfort. Sometimes powerful painkillers are prescribed. One of the most important steps in filling a prescription is to make sure you are aware of the potential benefits

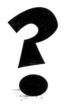

You've got health questions – I've got health answers.

How does the price of natural alternatives and remedies compare to over-the-counter or prescription drugs?

-They are most often a safer and less expensive...

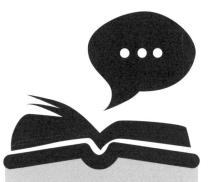

and risks of the drug you are about to take. Before you commit to a lifetime of medication or drug therapy you should spend some time researching the drug for both the positive and negative effects it will have on your health. It is important to make sure you are getting the treatment that is right for you. Too many people rely on drugs that may be unlikely to help. Drug labels should list potential side effects for the drug(s), and it is important to research and understand those adverse effects before you begin taking the drug(s).

A side effect is a secondary effect that occurs in addition to the desired therapeutic effect of a drug or medication. Usually this effect is undesirable. Side effects vary depending on a person's age, weight, gender and general health. They can occur during a regimen or manifest after the drug is discontinued.

Some adverse effects you might experience can cause mental, nervous system, immune system or gastrointestinal reactions. Mental reactions might include confusion, depression, hallucinations, memory loss, insomnia or impaired thinking. Nervous system reactions may include dizziness, falls, involuntary movements, numbness, tingling, and sexual dysfunction. Gastrointestinal reactions may include nausea, loss of appetite, diarrhea, abdominal pain, bleeding, bloating or constipation. Immune reactions may include allergic response, fatigue, susceptibility to infection, hives, rash, low white blood count.

Most adverse effects are linked specifically to a certain drug or type of drug. Some drugs prescribed for other health challenges may eventually cause nerve damage. For example a British medical journal recently reported that cholesterol lowering statin drugs could raise a person's risk of developing Type 2 diabetes by 9 percent. Statin cholesterol lowering drugs such as Lipitor, Crestor, Lescol, Zocor, Pravachol, Torvast, etc. may also been linked to nerve, brain, eye, liver and muscle damage, and can also cause peripheral neuropathy. Many users complain of muscle aches, fatigue, and pain. Patients who take Statins are also warned about the importance of being tested regularly to make sure liver enzymes are not abnormally high. There are a number of safe cholesterol management options found in health food stores.

You've got health questions – I've got health answers.

Tips to help you avoid adverse effects from over-the-counter drugs
- Don't take medicine with alcoholic drinks.
- Don't take a higher dose of the medicine than the label tells you to.
- Don't take the medicine more frequently than suggested.
- Make sure you know what ingredients the product contains and understand any warnings or possible adverse effects.
- Don't mix medicine into hot drinks unless the label tells you to.
- The heat may keep the drug from working as it should.
- Limit how often you use over the counter medications. Don't use them unless you really need them.

I'll be your designated driver on the highway to health.

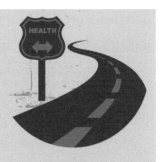

Some adverse effects associated with prescription drug use:

Acne
Addiction
Allergic reaction
Amnesia
Anemia
Anxiety
Birth defects
Bleeding of the
intestine
Bloating
Blood Clots
Blurred Vision
Breathing difficulties
Bruising
Cardiovascular disease
Chest Pain
Confusion
Constipation
Deafness
Death
Dementia
Depression
Diabetes
Diarrhea
Dizziness
Drowsiness
Dry Eyes

Dry Mouth
Edema
Erectile dysfunction
Facial Tics
Fatigue
Fever
Glaucoma
Hair loss
Headache
Heartburn
High Blood Pressure
Hives
Hyperglycemia
Hypoglycemia
Hypertension
Increased Appetite
Immune System
   Damage
Inflammation
Insomnia
Irregular Heartbeat
Itching
Jaundice
Joint Pain
Kidney failure
Lactic acidosis
Liver damage

Loss of Appetite
Loss of Libido
Low Blood Pressure
Miscarriage
Mood Swings
Mouth Sores
Muscle Pain
Nausea
Nervousness
Pain
Peripheral neuropathy
Rash
Restlessness
Seizures
Sensitivity to Light
Stomach Pain
Stroke
Suicide
Sweating
Tendon rupture
Thirst
Toxicity
Ulcers
Vomiting
Weight Gain
Weight Loss
Wheezing

Anti-anxiety drugs such as Cymbalta, also have adverse side effects such as nausea, abdominal pain and headaches.

Lyrica, Neurontin, Lamictal, Topamax, and other anticonvulsant drugs used to treat fibromyalgia and neuropathic pain, may increase a patient's risk of suicidal thoughts and behaviors.

Common Potential Side effects of Drugs such as these:

- Fatigue
- Drowsiness
- Mental and physical slowing or delays
- Nervousness
- Upper respiratory infection
- Coordination problems
- Confusion
- Difficulty with concentration
- Nausea
- Memory loss
- Language or speech problems
- Sinus infection
- Decreased sense of touch
- Mood problems
- Back pain
- Impotence

HEALTH OUTRAGE:

Unintentional drug poisoning death rates increased substantially in the United States during 1999-2004. This increase can primarily be attributed to increasing numbers of deaths associated with prescription opioids (which are types of painkillers such as OxyContin and Vicodin).

Source: CDC. "Unintentional Poisoning Deaths— United States, 1999 - 2004," 2007.

Other potential adverse side effects of drugs used to treat neuropathy include dizziness, sleepiness, edema, blurred vision, dry mouth, swelling of hands and feet, constipation, weight gain, difficulty with concentration. Often the side effects of these drugs may be worse than the nerve related concern itself. Research suggests that the evidence that anticonvulsants are effective for acute pain is limited, and that other interventions should be tried before turning to these types of drugs.

NSAIDs, Nonsteroidal anti-inflammatory drugs, include aspirin, ibuprofen and naproxen. Side effects include rash, nausea, heartburn, and ulcer disease. Muscle relaxants, which are used to treat muscle spasms, can cause drowsiness. Antidepressants can dull pain perception, but side effects include drowsiness, dry mouth and heart rhythm disturbances.

Fluoroquinolone antibiotics can cause adverse reactions involving many systems of the body including the peripheral nervous system. In 2004 the FDA mandated new warnings for the labeling of fluoroquinolone drugs to list the possibility of severe nerve injuries.

Anti-seizure drugs are often used to help control pain that is commonly caused by damaged nerves. However, their use is limited because of the severity of side effects. Possible side effects from anti-seizure drugs include: nausea, vomiting, liver damage, double vision, headache and loss of coordination.

Narcotics are often used to treat severe pain. They are powerful pain relievers and are generally used when other treatments fail. However, these drugs, including Morphine, and Oxycodone, have been linked to serious addiction and a dependency that causes significant disruption to a healthy life. Other side effects include sedation, confusion and nausea.

Neuroleptic psychiatric drugs may lead to diabetes.

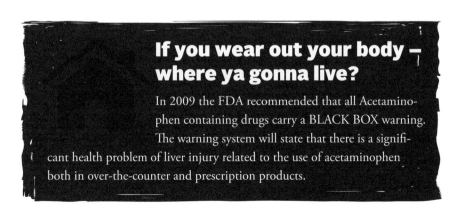

If you wear out your body – where ya gonna live?

In 2009 the FDA recommended that all Acetaminophen containing drugs carry a BLACK BOX warning. The warning system will state that there is a significant health problem of liver injury related to the use of acetaminophen both in over-the-counter and prescription products.

It is important to be aware that there may be a negative consequence attached to prescription drug use, and to use good judgment before committing to taking these drugs. And, in non-life-threatening or benign circumstances, why not consider safer options as outlined in this book?

If your current medication regimen isn't working for you, or if you are worried about possible adverse effects, make an appointment to speak to your physician. If you choose to discontinue a drug on your own be careful and withdraw slowly!

By the numbers

1.9 billion — Number of drugs ordered by a physician in one year.

47% — 47% of people used at least one prescription drug in the past month -CDC

6 — The average person over the age of 65 is taking 6 or more drugs.

136 — Over 136 drugs can cause cognitive impairment.

3.4 billion — Americans fill more than 3.4 billion prescriptions a year.

9.6 million — Almost 9.6 million older Americans experience negative side effects from their medications each year.

2 million — More than 2 million Americans are seriously injured by side effects each year.

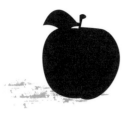

If you desire abundant health and wellness, you've come to the right place.

Ten Rules for Safer Drug Use

1. Make an appointment with your primary doctor to discuss all medications you currently take.

2. Ask your primary doctor to coordinate your care and drug use.

3. Make sure the drug therapy you are on is really needed.

4. If drug therapy is indicated, ask your doctor if it would be safe to start with a dose that is lower than the usual adult dose.

5. When adding a new drug, see if it is possible to discontinue another drug.

6. Always remember that stopping a drug is as important as starting it, ask your doctor before you discontinue drug use to make sure you are doing it correctly.

7. Find out if you are having any adverse drug reactions or side effects by reading information about the drug.

8. Before leaving you doctor's office or pharmacy, make sure the instructions for taking you medicine are clear to you.

9. Assume that any new symptom you develop after starting a new drug may be caused by the drug.

10. Discard all old drugs carefully.

Chapter Six
Safe and Effective Natural
REMEDIES

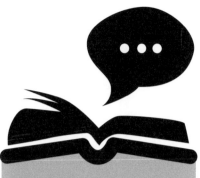

There is no such thing as a single cause of any health problem unless it happens to be an intended or stray bullet. We can only talk about cofactors, causative agents and life situations that interact with each other like pieces of a puzzle, and together promote a chain of events ending with a named set of symptoms and health problems including nerve related challenges.

Your body didn't come with an owner's manual, so I'm here for you.

The World Health Organization has stated that homeopathy is the second leading system of medicine for primary health care in the world, and is considered mainstream healthcare in Europe.

Since its inception 200 years ago, homeopathy has attracted support from European royalty, the educated elite and leading artists including Vincent van Gogh.

All disorders and health problems that happen to humans are multidimensional, because we, as humans, are multidimensional. Often modern medical theory is primarily interested in physical, chemical, and psycho-social elements. It may blame unsolved or misunderstood health problems on bad genes, bad viruses, bad bacteria, or any other number of factors.

Genes are always a factor of our health, but that is the only factor we can't do anything about. Genes represent approximately one third

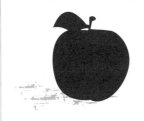

If you desire abundant health and wellness, you've come to the right place.

It is more important to know what sort of person has a disease than to know what sort of disease a person has.

–Hippocrates

of our predisposition and potential to encounter certain problem or disease. Whereas our lifestyle choices set the stage two thirds of the time for whether we are going to experience certain health challenges or not.

There are virtually thousands of cofactors, causative agents, and vectors that have a casual and/or direct relationship to poor immunity, poor health, toxic body burden, and poor thoughts that promote or perpetuate illness!

Try Something Different

It is hard not to suffer through life if you are in constant pain. Sometimes doing all that your healthcare provider suggests is still not enough. If you have not reached a state of wellbeing that you are happy with, don't be afraid to seek for more answers.

Sometimes the best remedy is a natural one. Take time to do something healthy for yourself. Improving your outlook on life goes a long way in improving your health. Take care of you —naturally and positively.

Taking care of your health at home can be accomplished easily if you know what to do.

Start by eating right. Healthy foods improve health. Add more fruits and vegetables to your diet. Include raw nuts and seeds. Choosing the right foods can give essential vitamins and nutrients that your body needs. Some nerve conditions and disorders will completely resolve and even disappear when a healthy diet is adhered to. Sometimes all it takes is making sure your body is properly absorbing the nutrients it needs.

Spend some time reading. Both the Internet and your local library are full of ideas on how to improve your health at home. If something is wrong with your health, do some research. Learn all you can about the subject. What do physicians suggest? How about researching some natural remedies? Taking time to research the facts will help you to become your own best advocate. Quality time spent researching could make a world of difference in your health.

Take some time for you. Remedies such as warm baths, saunas, steam rooms, and long walks can go a long way in improving overall health. Taking a nap, or catching up on sleep may be exactly what your body needs right now. Slow down. Also, don't forget to set aside time for exercise. Participate in a form of exercise you enjoy and stick with it.

Do Something Positive

Prioritize your health. Make it most important. Set aside time to do something positive for your health and wellbeing every single day.

Speaking about neuropathy Sue McLaughlin, RD, CDE, president of health care and education for the American Diabetes Association said, "You live with it every day, and you can do something positive about it daily, too." Here are some self-care tips you can try at home:

1. **Control Blood Sugar Levels.** "Controlling your sugar isn't just your No. 1 strategy; it's practically the whole top ten." (Sue McLaughlin) Studies show that keeping blood glucose levels close to normal can improve pain and stop ongoing damage.

2. **Prevent Neuropathic Pain With proper foot Care.** Clean and care for your feet. Wear comfortable shoes and socks. Cut your toenails strait across. Visit a DPM (Doctor of Podiatric Medicine) for foot care concerns and maintenance.

3. **Walk to Heal Damaged Nerves.** Exercise improves blood flow and can help nourish damaged nerves back to health.

4. **Warm Water Treatment.** Some people find that a regular warm bath provides some relief from mild nerve pain. Warm baths boost blood flow to the skin of the legs and feet.

5. **Vitamin B Complex May Help Nerve Pain.** The B vitamins are essential for nerve health and may help improve nerve pain. But do not take more than 50 milligrams a day.

6. **Capsaicin: The Hot Chili Pepper Treatment.** Capsaicin cream rubbed on skin can bring relief from nerve pain. Apply it three to four times a day.

7. **Less Beer for Less Pain.** Because high levels of alcohol are toxic to nerves, reducing the amount of alcohol you drink may help with nerve pain.

8. **Botanical Oils for Nerve Pain.** Botanical oils such as geranium oil, black cumin seed oil, nutmeg oil, helichrysum Immortelle, wintergreen, and lavender oil have shown to reduce the pain of neuralgia.

http://diabetes.webmd.com/features/peripheral-neuropathy-and-diabetes (Peripheral Neuropathy and Diabetes, by Matthew Hoffman, MD)

Healing Affirmations

Sometimes improving your health is as simple as changing the way you think. Affirmations are often described as the practice of positive thinking. Positive affirmations are short, positive statements that serve as self-nurturing beliefs. Affirmations can reprogram thought patterns, helping to change the way you think and also helping to change the way you feel about things. Affirmations can change the energy that flows through your body. Sometimes changing the way you think can reprogram your mind, removing

HEALTH ALTERNATIVE:

Some of the health benefits of positive thinking include:

*   Increased life span
*   Lower rates of depression
*   Lower levels of distress
*   Greater resistance to the common cold
*   Better psychological and physical well-being
*   Reduced risk of death from cardiovascular disease
*   Better coping skills during hardships and times of stress

http://www.mayoclinic.com/health/positive-thinking/SR00009

beliefs that may be sabotaging your health. Surrounding yourself with positive statements, affirmations and proverbs about good health can have a lasting effect on your health and outlook on life.

Affirmations:

I am strong and healthy.
I am full of energy and vitality.
My body repairs and heals itself quickly.
I feel healing with every breath.
I accept good health as natural for me.
I have control of my health and wellness.
I will enjoy good health today.
I am healthy and whole.

This is a place where like-minded people gather to get well.

"The introduction of homeopathy forced the old school doctor to stir around and learn something of a rational nature about his business. You may honestly feel grateful that homeopathy survived the attempts of allopaths (the orthodox physicians) to destroy it."

–Mark Twain

Homeopathy

One of the best ways to improve overall health is to learn more about natural healing. Homeopathy is a whole medical system that was developed over 200 years ago in Germany. The developer of this form of medicine was Samuel Christian Hahnemann, MD. It is used for both wellness and prevention, but can also be used to treat many diseases and conditions. One common principle behind homeopathy is that "like cures like." In other words, a disease can be cured by a substance that produces a similar symptom in a healthy person. This idea can be traced back to Hippocrates who was the first to use the law of similars in Western culture. Homeopathic researches have found that herbs taken in low dosages were capable of curing the same symptoms they produced when taken in high doses. For example, if you are sick you would take a medicine containing a diluted substance that would cause the same symptoms as your disease in a healthy person when given in full strength. This will stimulate the body to reverse the imbalance that is causing your symptoms.

Homeopathy believes that the lower the dose of the medication, the greater its effectiveness. Within the remedy the substance has left its imprint, or essence, which will stimulate the body to heal itself. Ho-

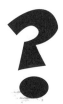
You've got health questions – I've got health answers.

"Homeopathy cures a larger percentage of cases than any other method of treatment and is beyond doubt safer and more economical and is the most complete medical science." –Mahatama Gandhi

meopaths are able to tailor treatments to each individual person. They look at health history, body type, and physical, mental, and emotional symptoms. Homeopathy follows the Hippocratic Tradition, first, do no harm.

Using natural substances that come from plants, minerals, or purified animal ingredients, the treatments are safe for people of all ages, even pregnant and nursing mothers. The substance is diluted in liquid repeatedly, and must be vigorously shaken with each dilution. Because the substance is very diluted it is extremely safe. Homeopaths do not treat the disease itself; rather, they treat the person. They believe that every symptom, whether physical, emotional, or mental combines together to represent a state of imbalance that is extremely specific to the individual. The solution is sought with this complete wellness in mind.

There are many safe and effective homeopathic medicines used in treatment for nerve pain and neuralgia. Used at full strength some of these remedies could prove life threatening and even fatal. These remedies must be diluted by a Homeopath to ensure safe use.

Aconitum napellus:

Aconitum napellus is a plant considered to be of therapeutic importance. If you touch juice from the root to your lip, the juice produces a feeling of numbness and tingling. The traditional medicine of Asia has used aconite for many years. It is known to first stimulate the nerve and then numb the nerve to the sensations of pain, touch and temperature. Great caution must be required so as not to use a dangerous dose. Aconite is one of the most frequently used remedies, and is almost specific for facial neuralgias. When mixed for neuralgia, it is often used in higher potencies. It has an effective action on the trigeminal nerve.

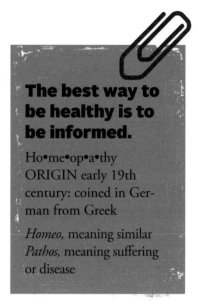

The best way to be healthy is to be informed.

Ho•me•op•a•thy
ORIGIN early 19th century: coined in German from Greek
Homeo, meaning similar
Pathos, meaning suffering or disease

Arnica montana:

Arnica Montana is a flowering plant from Europe and has been used medicinally for many years. Contact with the plant can cause skin irritation. The roots have some anti-inflammatory effect. It is often used in liniment and ointment preparations. It may help with deep muscle pain.

Hypericum perforatum:

Also known as St. John's Wort, Hypericum is often used for nerve injuries. It has shown to help remedy pain especially for areas rich in nerve endings.

Cimicifuga racemosa:

Cimicifuga is a remedy for afflictions of the nervous system. It is used as a remedy for sharp pains.

Ruta graveolens:

Ruta graveolens is a herb that was first used in European folk medicine. It is often made into an ointment and used externally against

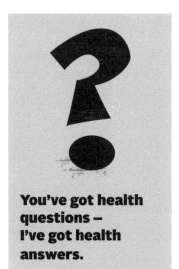

You've got health questions – I've got health answers.

Can homeopathy really make a difference?

The Bristol Homeopathic Hospital carried out a study published in November 2005 of 6500 patients receiving homeopathic treatment. 70% showed an overall improvement in health. *(http://news.bbc.co.uk/1/hi/england/...).*

neuralgia. It can be used to help sciatica or to help with stiffness in the muscles.

Spigelia anthelmia:

Spigelia is a tropical weed and exerts a powerful action on the nervous system. It is commonly used for conditions that affect the nerves themselves. It is beneficial for sensory nerves and helps with sticking, tearing and burning pains, especially pains that are aggravated by motion. If the body is sensitive to touch, this is the right remedy.

Colocynthis:

Native of Northern Africa, the colocynth is an annual plant that can be used for visceral pain. If the pain is cutting, darting, and cramping colocynth should be used. Colocynth is used for neuralgias that are recent, not chronic and is particularly valuable in neuralgic pains. The neuralgia must be a nervous type, not inflammatory.

Belladonna:

Belladonna is a perennial plant native to Europe, North Africa and Asia. It has a long history of medicinal use. Belladonna is a toxic plant, and ingestion of a single leaf can be fatal. It is used homeopathically for infra-orbital neuralgia that is accompanied with an increase of tears and saliva. It can block the neurotransmitters in the central and peripheral nervous system. Belladonna is used if there are violent pains that increase towards evening, and are made worse from noise, motion, chewing or cold air.

Arsenicum album:

Arsenicum album is a substance derived from the metallic element arsenic. It is considered one of the fifteen most important remedies in homeopathy. Arsenicum is often used to treat ailments that are characterized by burning pain. It is especially effective if the affection is purely nervous. It can be used for intermitting burning, stinging, and restlessness. Its effect is rapid. Some say Arsenicum quiets nervous pain better than any other medicine.

Platina:

Platinum was discovered in South America in the 18th century. It is used to make jewelry. In homeopathy it is most often used for ailments of the nervous system in which there is a numbness of the skin. Platinum should be used when there is numbness and constrictive pain that becomes worse at night and with rest. If the pains are cramping and cause numbness and tingling while increasing and decreasing gradually, platinum is the right remedy.

Sulphur:

Sulphur may be used as a remedy as a homeopathy nerve pain reliever. It is often used for itching and burning pains.

Phosphorus:

Ailments helped by phosphorus are characterized by burning pain.

Thallium:

Thallium is helpful for spasmodic, shooting pains common with neuralgia. It may be helpful with numbness of lower limbs. Electric shocks and pains may also be helped by Thallium.

Mezereum:

The dried bark of the mezereum has been used to treat disease for many years. It is often used for skin disorders. It can help sooth the severe stabbing pain caused by neuralgia. This remedy should be used if there is a numbness remaining after the attack. It is often used with shingles.

Verbascum:

Verbascum is a weedy plant that has astringent properties. It can be used topically for a variety of skin problems. Verbascum is used for pressure and pain involving the upper jaw, especially if it is worse on the right side. It has been known to help with severe cases. If the neuralgia is not confined to the face only, but extends to the neck and shoulders verbascum should be considered.

Magnesia phosphorica:

Magnesia phosphoricum has an excellent clinical record. This remedy often cures diseases that are found in the nerve fiber cells or in the muscular tissue. Pains that are cramping, darting or lightning-like respond to Magnesia phosphorica. It is used when the pains are intermitting and relieved by warmth.

Calcarea carbonica:

Calcera carbonica is one of the most commonly used remedies. It comes from the inner lining in shells, and is ground into a fine powder. It is commonly used to treat ailments that are aggravated by cold weather. This remedy helps if nerve pain comes from an aversion to cold air.

Lycopodium:

Lycopodium is a creeping plant that has a medicinal effect on soft tissues, joints, bones, blood vessels, the liver and the heart. It has been used for treatment with joint pain and muscle cramps.

Ambra Grisea :

Ambra Grisea is a waxy substance produced in the digestive system of a sperm whale. It is found floating upon the sea or in the sand near the coast line. It is considered an aphrodisiac. Ambra Grisea is known to help cramps in thighs, calves and feet and contraction of hamstrings. It also may be used for paralytic weakness with numbness.

Kalium Phosphate

Kalium Phosphate is a biochemic salt that is an essential factor of the human nervous system. It is important to the brains ability to concentrate. It is helpful for many neurological disorders.

Causticum

Causticum is remedy derived from quicklime otherwise known as Calcium oxide or potassium bisulphate, and was invented by Samuel Hahnemann. It's used for left-sided sciatica with numbness, paralysis of single parts, and Bell's palsy. Cauticum can also help with dull or tearing pain in hands and arms, numbness or loss of sensation in hands, stiffness between shoulders, dull pain in nape of neck.

Ferrum Phosphoricum

This remedy, derived from iron phosphate, can be ffective in the first stages of inflammation. Ferrum phosphoricum cal also help with stiff neck, crick in back, rheumatic pain in shoulder, pain extend to chest and wrist, and facial neuralgia.

Rhus Toxicodendron

Also known as poison ivy, Rhus Toxicodendron is used to relieve stiffness, painful muscles that seize up with rest but loosen up with exercise and heat, stiffness in lower back, numbness in arms and legs, and sciatica.

Sanguinaria

Sanguinaria is indicated for burning sensations in palms, toes and soles, neuralgia including pain that extends in all directions from upper jaw, right sided neuritis, periodical sick headache, pain that begins in occipital, spreads upward, and settles over eyes especially right, and rheumatism of right shoulder, left hip joint and nape of neck.

Silicea

Derived from silica or pur flint, Silicea can help with pain in coccyx, sciatica, pains through hips, legs and feet. cramps in calves and soles, loss of power in legs, pain in knee as if tightly bound, pain beneath toes and sore soles.

Homeopathic remedies should be considered if you are experiencing strong attacks of nerve pain. These remedies are specific to certain kinds of pain and will help with fiery pain, tearing sensations, electric shock, shooting or sharp pains, lightening quick cramps, stabbing pains, numbness, tingling, and sensitivity to being touched. A person educated in homeopathy can help you decide which remedy will work best for your condition.

Replace something you already do with something better:

_____

_____

_____

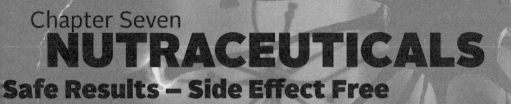

Chapter Seven
NUTRACEUTICALS
Safe Results – Side Effect Free

A nutraceutical is a food or food substance that provides health and medicinal benefits. These are foods that have demonstrated a physiological benefit or provide protection against chronic disease. Nearly two-thirds of the American population takes at least one type of nutraceutical. In fact, the nutraceutical industry in the US totals about $86 billion a year. One of the reasons nutraceuticals are becoming so prevalent is because they provide health benefits without side effects.

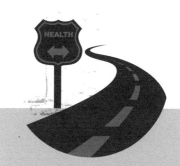

I'll be your designated driver on the highway to health.

"The doctor of the future will no longer treat the human frame with drugs, but rather will cure and prevent disease with nutrition."

–Thomas Edison

It was Hippocrates who first suggested that people should "Let food be thy medicine." Research suggests that he may have been right. Food science is beginning to show that there is more to food than just its taste, texture and nutritional value, science is now measuring food for probiotics, antioxidants and more. Certain nutraceuticals have actually been tested by the US Food and Drug Administration and have been deemed appropriate for use in the prevention of select ailments. Others are currently in the process. Nutraceuticals can do more than just supplement your diet; they can also help with disease prevention and treatment.

Nutraceuticals can be defined as nutrients, or foods with nutritional functions that include vitamins, minerals, amino acids and fatty acids, herbs or botanical products, and dietary supplements such as probiotics, antioxidants and enzymes. Nutraceuticals can be taken orally or used topically.

The most common nutrients used as nutraceuticals are vitamins and minerals. Take a moment to look at the chart below and see the health benefits of different common vitamins.

Vitamin A	Required for normal vision, gene expression, reproduction, embryonic development and immune function. May aid in the prevention and treatment of certain cancers. May also aid in the treatment of certain skin disorders. (Liver, dairy products, fish, darkly colored fruits and leafy vegetables.)
Vitamin B1	Also known as Thiamine, Vitamin B1 is highly involved in nervous system and muscle functioning, including the flow of electrolytes in and out of nerve and muscle cells. Very little thiamine is stored in the body, and depletion can occur in less than 14 days. Healthy sources of thiamine include brown rice, fish, egg yolks, legumes, peas, peanuts, poultry, whole grains, wheat germ, poultry, broccoli, Brussels sprouts, most nuts, spirulina, brewers yeast, oatmeal, watercress and prunes. *NOTE: Allithiamine (Thiamine tetrahytdrofurfurly disulfide) is a lipid-soluble form of Vitamin B1. It is typically more easily absorbed than other forms of B1. The functions of vitamin B1 also include carbohydrate metabolism, nerve conduction and transmissions, energy production and oxygen metabolism.*
Vitamin B6	Also known as pyridoxine, Vitamin B6 is required by the nervous system, and is needed for normal brain function and for the synthesis of the nucleic acids RNA and DNA, which contain the genetic instructions for the reproduction of all cells and for normal cellular growth. A deficiency can affect the peripheral nerves, skin, mucous membranes, and the blood cell system. Healthy sources of pyridoxine include brewer's yeast, fish, chicken, eggs, spinach, peas, wheat germ, walnuts, sunflower seeds, carrots, broccoli, corn, brown rice, whole grains, cabbage, soybeans, tempeh, cantaloupe, and rice bran.

Vitamin B12	Also known as cobalamin, Vitamin B12is required for proper digestion, absorption of foods, the synthesis of protein, and the metabolism of carbohydrates and fats. Additionally, vitamin B12 prevents nerve damage and promotes normal growth and development by maintaining the fatty insulation that cover and protect nerve endings. *NOTE: Methylcobalamin is the "active" and preferred form of cobalamin when it especially concerns nerve function and repair. Your liver has to transform regular vitamin B12 (cyanocobalamin) into methylcobalamin. Sources include: Brewer's yeast, eggs, dairy products, seafood, soybeans, sea vegetables, fortified cereals, meat, and poultry.)*
Vitamin C	Also known as ascorbic acid, Vitamin C is an antioxidant that is required for tissue growth and repair. It is essential in the formation of collagen and promotes healing. Vitamin C can be found in citrus fruits, berries, green vegetables, avocados, onions, black currants, tomatoes, potatoes, brussel sprouts, cauliflower, peppers, broccoli, strawberries, cabbage and spinach.
Vitamin D	Vitamin D maintain serum calcium and phosphorus concentrations. It can be found in fish liver oils, fortified eggs and milk products, and fortified cereals.
Vitamin E	An antioxidant which helps to form blood cells and boost immune system, Vitamin E can be found in vegetable oils, unprocessed cereal grains, nuts, fruits, vegetables, and meats.
Vitamin K	Involved in blood clotting and bone metabolism, Vitamin K is found in green vegetables including spinach, salad greens, broccoli, brussel sprouts, and cabbage.
Pantothenic Acid	Coenzyme in fatty acid metabolism, Pantothenic Acid is found in chicken, beef, potatoes, oats, cereals, tomato products, liver, kidney, yeast, egg yolk, broccoli, and whole grains.
Niacin	Coenzyme in many biological reduction and oxidation reactions, Niacin is required for energy metabolism. It can be found in meat, fish, poultry, enriched and whole-grain bread products, and fortified ready-to-eat cereals.
Folate	Coenzyme in the metabolism of nucleic and amino acids, Folate prevents megaloblastic anemia. Folate can be found in enriched nriched cereal grains, dark leafy vegetables, enriched and whole-grain breads and bread products, and fortified and ready-to-eat cereals.

Minerals and Herbs also play a role in keeping the body healthy and prevention against disease. For example, magnesium can be used for healthy nerve and muscle function, and ginger can be used to combat dizziness. Studies are being done that allow science to combine food ingredients rich in nutraceuticals. These food products are fortified with active ingredients that maximize health potential.

Some nutraceuticals have shown to be beneficial for nerve conditions. Many other nutraceuticals show an ability to help calm symptoms associated with nerve disorders. There are positive findings that suggest the importance of increasing the uptake of antioxidants to improve health in the central nervous system. Research shows that the health benefits from nutraceuticals are making them a powerful instrument not only in maintaining health, but also in helping to act against chronic diseases.

Here are some nutraceuticals and their benefits:

Alpha lipoic acid:

Alpha lipoic acid is an antioxidant that is found inside every cell of the body. Its ability to kill free radicals may help protect against nerve damage and reduce tingling, burning, pain, and numbness. Alpha lipoic acid has shown to enhance glucose transport and utilization, and may improve insulin sensitivity in Type 2 diabetics. It has also been shown to reduce symptoms of diabetic peripheral neuropathy and improve cardiac autonomic nerve dysfunction.

Benfotiamine:

Benfotiamine is a derivative of thiamine and was developed in Japan. It has been used to treat patients with nerve damage and nerve pain, alcoholic neuropathy, sciatica, and other painful nerve conditions. Benfotiamine is one of the most well-researched alternative options for the treatment of Peripheral neuropathy.

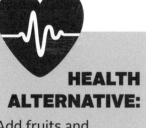

HEALTH ALTERNATIVE:

Add fruits and vegetables to your diet!

Only about one-fourth of U.S. adults eat the recommended five or more servings of fruits and vegetables each day.

Preventing Obesity and Chronic Diseases Through Good Nutrition and Physical Activity, Centers for Disease Control and Prevention, August 2003. www.cd.gov

Methylcobalamin:

Methylcobalamin is a form of vitamin B12 and is often used in the treatment of peripheral neuropathy and diabetic neuropathy. It has been shown to relieve symptoms in the legs, such as paresthesia, burning pains and heaviness. Methylcobalamin has also proved beneficial in nerve regeneration. It has been shown to be highly effective and safe for treating the symptoms of diabetic neuropathy.

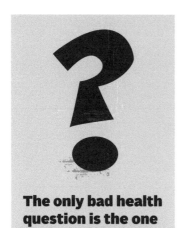

Passion Flower:

Passion flower when used in folk medicine is thought to be a calming herb. It is valued for its analgesic properties. It has a sedative and antispasmodic action and can calm the nerves and lessen pain. It has been used in the treatment of neuralgia, shingles, sciatica, and with muscle pains and twitches.

Myo-inositol:

Myo-inositol is found in many foods including bran, nuts, beans and fruit. It has been used in the treatment of diabetic neuropathy.

Astragalus membranaceus:

Also known as AM extract. Can be a potential nerve growth-promoting factor.

Goto Kola:

A medicinal herb used for thousands of years to heal wounds and as a nerve tonic. Studies show that Goto Kola may be useful for accelerating repair of damaged neurons.

Velvet antler:

Velvet antler is dried and used for a wide variety of health purposes. It is known as an anti-inflammatory and also as a pro-growth agent. It may help promote nerve survival and development.

Pyridoxine:

Pyridoxine is one of the compounds in vitamin B6. It is often used to treat or prevent nerve problems such as peripheral neuropathy or other central nervous system challenges.

Betaine HCL:

Taking betaine can aid in protein digestion. One of the benefits of betaine hydrochloride is to protect against diabetic neuropathy.

Magnesium:

Magnesium is a chemical element. Magnesium ions are essential to the basic chemistry of life. Low levels of magnesium in the body have been associated with the development of a number of human illnesses. Magnesium helps to keep nerves relaxed. A magnesium deficiency can trigger muscle tension, cramps and spasms.

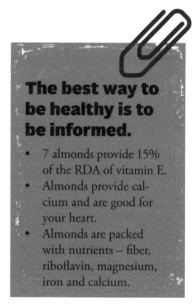

The best way to be healthy is to be informed.

- 7 almonds provide 15% of the RDA of vitamin E.
- Almonds provide calcium and are good for your heart.
- Almonds are packed with nutrients — fiber, riboflavin, magnesium, iron and calcium.

Vitamin D:

Vitamin D is obtained from sun exposure, food and supplements. In the United States milk, yogurt, and bread are all fortified with vitamin D. Vitamin D is known to aid in nerve growth. One study published in the Archives of Internal Medicine found that vitamin D supplementation cut nerve pain from diabetic neuropathy almost in half.

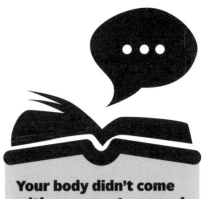

Your body didn't come with an owner's manual, so I'm here for you.

5 foods that can lower your cholesterol and protect your heart:
- oatmeal
- almonds
- salmon
- olive oil
- orange juice fortified with sterols

Evening Primrose Oil:

Evening Primrose is a flowering plant native to North and South America. Evening Primrose Oil is said to possess astringent and sedative properties. It may be used as a sedative pain-killer.

Fish Oil:

Fish oil has been known to block the production of inflammatory chemicals called cytokines and leukotrienes in the body. These chemicals are responsible for conditions such as rheumatoid arthritis, Crohn's disease, gout and sinusitis. Eating three grams of fish fats a day may help with joint pain, inflammation, and morning stiffness. Some patients have been able to discontinue use of anti-inflammatory medication after a regimen of fish oil use (See page 159 - Nordic Naturals).

Tart Cherries:

Researches at MSU have discovered that eating 20 tart cherries may relieve pain better than aspirin. The cherries may also exhibit antioxidant properties. In fact, daily consumption of cherries may help to reduce pain related to inflammation, arthritis and gout.

Noni fruit:

Studies done on Morinda citrifolia, a tropical plant with a long tradition of medicinal use in Polynesia, have shown that the fruit possesses a strong analgesic effect. Preparations of noni fruit can be effective in decreasing pain. Tahiti Trader manufactures a variety of high potency Noni juice products.

Tumeric:

Turmeric contains the compound curcumin, a powerful painkiller that has been known to block inflammatory proteins and suppress inflammation. It can be used in place of NSAIDs without any side effects to the heart, liver, stomach, and kidneys. Curcumin may ease chronic pain by stopping the neurotransmitter substance P from sending its pain signals to the brain. Curcumin also decreases inflammation.

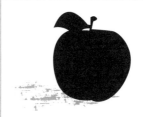

If you desire abundant health and wellness, you've come to the right place.

An apple a day will give you...
- Pectin, a soluble fiber than can lower blood cholesterol and glucose levels.
- Vitamin C – a powerful antioxidant

One of the most potent curcumin products on the market today, is Curamin by; EuroPharma

Thiamine:

Thiamine is also known as vitamin B1. Insufficient intake of thiamine affects the peripheral nervous system. Yeast is the best source of thiamine. Whole grains also contain thiamine. Thiamine aids the nervous system and is essential for the transmission of certain types of nerve signals. Poor memory, muscle weakness, nerve tingling, burning and numbness are all signs of thiamin deficiency. Increased levels of thiamine in the blood stream are effective in reducing and reversing nerve pain. Thiamine is also needed by the body to heal nerve damage.

Riboflavin:

Riboflavin, also known as vitamin B, is found in milk, cheese, leafy green vegetables, legumes, tomatoes and almonds. It is essential for normal nerve function.

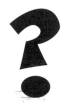

You've got health questions – I've got health answers.

Blueberries can help prevent chronic diseases, improve short-term memory and promote healthy aging.

Folic acid:

Folic acid, also known as vitamin B9, is crucial for proper brain function. Leafy vegetables, fruits, beans, peas, and grain products are rich sources of folate.

Acetyl L-carnitine:

Acetyl L-carnitine naturally occurs in plants and animals. It is a powerful antioxidant, and has shown to be neuro-protective. This supplement is often used as a treatment for nerve pain, particularly if the pain results from diabetes.It may be useful in treating peripheral nerve injury. ALC has an antinociceptive effect making it useful in preventing the development neuropathic pain. ALC has also been known to improve the function of peripheral nerves by reducing sensory neuron loss and promoting nerve regeneration.

Biotin:

Biotin is a B-complex vitamin and may be helpful in maintaining a steady blood sugar level. It also can play a role in preventing neuropathy and may reduce both numbness and tingling.

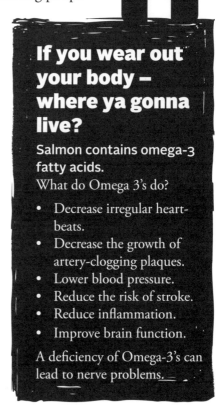

If you wear out your body – where ya gonna live?

Salmon contains omega-3 fatty acids.
What do Omega 3's do?

- Decrease irregular heartbeats.
- Decrease the growth of artery-clogging plaques.
- Lower blood pressure.
- Reduce the risk of stroke.
- Reduce inflammation.
- Improve brain function.

A deficiency of Omega-3's can lead to nerve problems.

Botanical Plants:

There are also several botanical plant species that have proven helpful with inflammation-related ailments such as muscle swelling and nerve related pains. These species include:

Bombax ceiba

Canarium strictum

Chloranthus erectus

Xanthium indicum

Lycopodium clavatum

Coleus blumei

Batrachospermum atrum

Chlorella vulgaris

Marchantia palmata

Marchantia polymorpha

Eria pannea

Sterculia villosa

Alpinia galanga

Probiotics

Some species of friendly bacteria also known as probiotics in the gastrointestinal system manufacture vitamins from the B group – which are difficult to obtain from food and cannot be manufactured by humans. A healthy intestinal flora is important in the production of nerve growth and protecting vitamins B-3, B6, B12, and folic acid. As well as their helpful effects in maintaining an optimum digestive pH, supporting regularity, balancing hormones, helping to digest food, detoxify harmful substances, and stimulating the immune system, friendly gut bacteria are essential for general health and longevity. Unfortunately, usage of antibiotics, steroid drugs, synthetics hormone replacement, chlorinated water, processed foods, food poisoning, influenza, and stress can all harm our intestines ability to maintain health friendly bacteria and therefore, potential inhibit the ability to make nerve protecting B vitamins. One of the best probiotic and prebiotic supplements on the market today, is Dr. Ohirra's Probiotics 12 Plus.

Vitamin C

Vitamin C is considered an antioxidant required for hundreds of important bodily functions including, but not limited to; tissue growth and repair. Because the human body cannot manufacture vitamin C, it must be obtained through the diet (primarily fruits and vegetables) or via nutritional supplementation. However, most people consuming the SAD (Standard American Diet) fail to obtain the necessary servings of foods containing vitamin C, multiple supplemental doses of this important nutrient may be necessary. And, because some people are sensitive to acidic forms of vitamin C such as ascorbic acid, esterified vitamin C, or Ester-C by American Health is an excellent choice. This form of nonacidic vitamin C is gentle on the stomach and therefore may be taken in higher doses without causing diarrhea and other undesirable provocations. Additionally, Ester-C enters the blood stream and tissues four times faster than typical forms of vitamin C.

Chapter Eight
Topical Nerve
HELPERS

Topical treatments, like creams, lotions and gels, may help to ease nerve pain. They often work the best when used directly on the skin over the specific areas that are painful. Some nutraceuticals can be used topically to help promote optimal health. Topical creams can include ingredients that work as an anesthetic, numbing the pain in the area where they are applied. Others have analgesic effects, helping to control the pain and stimulate circulation. Topical treatments containing capsaicin, a painkiller that is found in chili peppers have proven to be effective. Often botanical oils are used. One of the best benefits of a topical treatment is that it can be used precisely where you need to find relief.

Listed below are some nutraceuticals that can be used topically, they exhibit properties conducive to promoting nerve health:

Topical Nutraceuticals

Nutmeg is a spice that was used by the Chinese for its medicinal properties. They discovered its use as an appetite stimulant, an anti-nausea agent, an inflammatory agent, and as a digestive stimulant.

Nutmeg can relax the muscles and sedate the body. It can also be used for acute and chronic nerve related disorders.

Eugenol, a phenylpropene obtained from the essential oils of clove and basil possesses analgesic effects. It has been shown to reduce neuronal excitability.

Lavender has been used medicinally for more than 2500 years. Lavender essential oils may provide relief from pain particularly in muscles.

Black Pepper is a powerful warming agent. Its therapeutic properties include analgesic, antiseptic, antitoxic and antispasmodic. It is extremely beneficial for aches, pains, muscle stiffness and even temporary paralysis. It is effective at stimulating the circulation and dilating blood vessels.

Peppermint oil, native of the Mediterranean, has been used for centuries for relief from nerve related issues. Peppermint can suppress pain, and is also used to fight mental fatigue and improve concentration. It can relieve pain in cases of neuralgia and muscle pain. It has a cooling action on the skin and is used to relieve skin irritations and itchiness.

Wintergreen was used by American Indians to treat back pain, rheumatism, fever and headaches. It has been used in traditional medicine as an analgesic, astringent and topical rubefacient and offers pain relief, helps constricts body tissues, and improves circulation. Wintergreen oil has a history of use as a pain reliever.

St. John Wort contains hypericin with anti-inflammatory properties. It was used historically to relieve nerve pain especially pain resulting from injury, strain, and shingles. It is particularly soothing to inflamed nerves, which makes it helpful for cases of neuralgia and sciatica.

Capsicum is a pepper native to America. Capsicum can dramatically reduce chronic nerve pain. When used as a lotion or cream and applied to the skin is has been known to relieve the pain of shingles and other nerve related issues.

Dimethyl sulfoxide (DMSO) is a by-product of the wood industry is known for its ability to ease pain. It has been used most widely as a topical analgesic. It also has anti-inflammatory and antioxidant properties.

Olive oil contains a natural chemical that influences the same biochemical pathway as ibuprofen and other non-steroidal anti-inflammatory drugs (NSAIDs). Research studies have shown that 50 grams of extra-virgin olive oil was comparable to about 10 per cent of the ibuprofen dose recommended for adult pain relief. Regular olive oil consumption can have lasting inflammatory effects.

White willow bark is an effective fever reducer and is capable of providing all of the pain relieving benefits of aspirin. It has been known to decrease pain by blocking the production of inflammatory prostaglandins. Studies have shown the white willow bark may provide relief to toothache, backache, headache, or even arthritis. Used to treat pain and inflammation since the ancient time of Egypt and Greece, willow bark has been shown to reduce fever and inflammation. Willow bark exhibits antioxidant, fever-reducing, antiseptic, and immune-boosting properties.

MSM (methyl-sulphonyl-methane) is a sulphur compound with anti-inflammatory, anti-spasmodic and analgesic properties. It has also been known to inhibit the transmission of pain impulses. It is available both as a dietary supplement and as a cream for topical application.

Glucosamine and Chondroitin are nutritional supplements that have been known to reduce pain in the joints. Glucosamine is commonly used in Europe as a painkiller. The supplements combined may also be effective in topical use.

Boswellia The acids founding Boswellia decrease the production of inflammatory compounds. It has shown to be helpful with pain, swelling and morning stiffness. Boswellia is known for its affect on the body to promote healthy inflammation response, reducing pain. This important botanical may also be used topically.

Devil's claw, native to South Africa is known for alleviating back pain and arthritis. It is known to have analgesic and anti-inflammatory effects.

Camphor is a white, crystalline substance that is extracted from the wood of an evergreen tree. It is available as an oil, ointment, salve and soap. Camphor has several health benefits. It can act as an effective anti-inflammatory by numbing the peripheral sensory nerves. It has been shown to offer relief from neuralgia, arthritis and back pain.

Anti-inflammatory Herbs

Link Matricaria recutita (German Chamomile): Known for its sedative and spasmolytic properties, chamomile also possesses anti-inflammatory activities. Because of its ability to penetrate intact skin deeply and exert an anti-inflammatory effect, chamomile is often used topically.

Zingiber officinale (Ginger): Ginger posseses anti-inflammatory benefits along with antitumor and antiproliferative properties. This herb may help to alleviate muscle strains.

Rosemary Extract is often used as a topical remedy for joint or musculoskeletal pain. It is known for its powerful ability to relieve muscle pains, sore muscles, headaches, rheumatism and arthritis.

Glycyrrhiza glabra (Licorice): Licorice has long been used in patients with high blood pressure, cardiac diseases, or liver cirrhosis. It contains a compound with anti-inflammatory activity.

Arnica montana (Arnica): Commonly used to treat bruises and swelling, this herb is also thought to possess anti-inflammatory properties. Internal use is safe when taken in a homeopathic diluted remedy, but Arnica can also be used topically to fight inflammation. This herb known for its ability to soothe sore muscles and inflammation.

Other herbs known to have anti-inflammatory activities include:

Hamamelis virginiana (witch hazel)

Echinacoside (echinacea)

Ananas comosus (pineapple)

Chapter Nine
Special Foods For
NERVES

Listed in this chapter you will find different kinds of food that promote nerve health. Research has shown that nutrition can have impact on healing and may facilitate the healing process. Nutritious foods and supplements have been shown to have many positive benefits when used to help treat the nervous system.

If you suffer from a nerve condition, are experiencing nerve pain or damage, or if you simply want healthier nerves consider adding these foods to your diet.

I'll be your designated driver on the highway to health.

1 Teaspoon of lemon juice in water can alkalinize the acidic buildup around your nerves and remove it from your body.

Vitamin B Complex:

A deficiency of vitamin B12 can often cause or worsen nerve pain. The Vitamin B Complex is highly involved in nervous system and muscle functioning, including the flow of electrolytes in and out of nerve and muscle cells. It aids the nervous system and is essential for the transmission of certain types of nerve signals. Poor memory, muscle weakness, nerve tingling, burning and numbness are all signs of vitamin B deficiency. Vitamin B is effective in reducing and reversing nerve pain, and is also needed by the body to heal nerve damage. It is essential for normal nerve function and can play a role in preventing neuropathy. Vitamin B may reduce both numbness and tingling.

Top 10 Food Sources for Vitamin B6

- Ready to eat cereal, 100% fortified
- Potato
- Banana
- Garbanzo beans
- Chicken breast
- Pork Loin
- Sunflower seeds
- Spinach
- Tomato Juice
- Avocado

Top 18 Healthy Food Sources for Vitamin B12

- Tempeh
- Miso
- Shoyu
- Tamari
- Sweeds
- Algae
- Nori
- Spirulina
- Fermented Soya
- Egg
- Nutritional yeast (Saccharomyces cervisiae)
- Ready to eat cereal, 100% fortified
- Trout
- Poulty
- Salmon
- Beef
- Yogurt
- Swiss Cheese

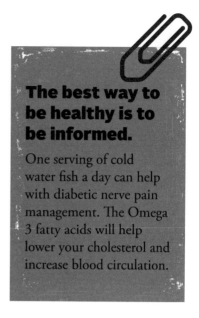

The best way to be healthy is to be informed.

One serving of cold water fish a day can help with diabetic nerve pain management. The Omega 3 fatty acids will help lower your cholesterol and increase blood circulation.

Magnesium

Magnesium helps to keep nerves relaxed. A magnesium deficiency can trigger muscle tension, cramps and spasms. Magnesium can also help fight muscle weakness. A deficiency of Magnesium may lead to irritability and even mental derangement.

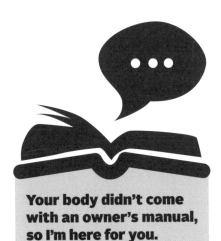

Your body didn't come with an owner's manual, so I'm here for you.
A small amount of walnuts or almonds can act as a great muscle relaxer that works quickly.

Top 10 Food Sources for Magnesium

- Halibut
- Almonds
- Cashews
- Soybeans
- Spinach
- Potato
- Peanuts, Peanut butter
- Yogurt
- Rice
- Avocado

Vitamin D

Vitamin D is known to aid in nerve growth. One study published in the Archives of Internal Medicine found that vitamin D supplementation cut nerve pain from diabetic neuropathy almost in half.

Top 10 Food Sources for Vitamin D

- Salmon
- Shrimp
- Cow's milk
- Cod
- Egg
- Herring
- Tofu
- Sardine
- Halibut
- Mushrooms

Omega 3

Omega 3 fatty acids help to reduce inflammation. They are important for brain memory and performance. A deficiency of fatty acids can lead to vision and nerve problems. One of the best supplement manufacturers for Omega 3 is Nordic Naturals.

Top 15 Food Sources for Omega 3 fatty acids

- Flaxseeds
- Cloves
- Walnuts
- Oregano
- Anchovies
- Arctic Char
- Salmon
- Sardine
- Halibut
- Herring
- Cauliflower
- Mustard seeds
- Cabbage
- Broccoli
- Brussels Sprouts
- Nordic Naturals-Utimate Omega

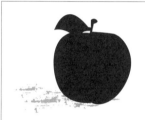

If you desire abundant health and wellness, you've come to the right place.

One serving of fresh walnuts will help control diabetic nerve pain.

Decrease or eliminate the following:

- Margarine
- Vegetable shortening
- Fried foods
- Partially hydrogenated fats
- Dairy products
- Vegetable oils
- Refined sugars
- Coffee
- Alcohol
- Soda pop

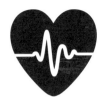

HEALTH ALTERNATIVE:

Anti-inflammatory Diet Tips

Over all, when you are choosing anti-inflammatory foods to help reduce your inflammation and pain, choose fresh foods instead of heavily processed foods. Here are some tips:

- Breakfast could be oatmeal quinoa, amaranth, or millet served with fresh berries and walnuts, with coconut, hemp, cashew or almond milk.

- Snack on whole organic fruits, nuts, seeds, and fresh vegetables throughout the day instead of cookies and candy.

- Eat more omega rich cold water fish such as wild salmon, sardines, herring,etc. and less fatty red meat.

- Stay away from deep fried foods and bake or stir fry your meals instead.

- Choose organic green, orange, purple and yellow vegetables for your side dishes. Drink plenty of purified water, fresh 100% fruit and vegetable juices, herbal teas and green tea.

- Use spices including ginger, tumeric, garlic, onions and cumin.

Replace something you already do with something better:

_____

_____

_____

Chapter Ten

Good Body Structure + Mobility
= BETTER
NERVE FUNCTION

Important Exercises for Nerve Health

Doctors are now advising that the estimated 20 million people in the US who suffer from peripheral neuropathy should participate in low-impact exercise. In fact, a study published in The Journal of Diabetes Complications in 2006 stated that there were significant benefits of exercise in controlling peripheral neuropathy. The research showed that exercise slowed the worsening of the nerve damage.

Some ideas for low-impact exercise are swimming, yoga, walking or cycling. The American Diabetes Association suggests that you should participate in some form of exercise or activity for a minimum of 30 minutes, 5 days a week. Walking, stretching, tai chi and pilates are all low-impact exercises that can be of great benefit to your health.

Yoga is a discipline that uses breath control, meditation and body postures. It has been shown to have substantial health benefits. A regular regime can increase your flexibility and stretch your muscles releasing the lactic acid that causes stiffness, tension and pain. Yoga can improve your muscle tone and your strength. It will benefit your posture and improve your breathing. Most people notice that they are less stressed and feel more calm after this type of exercise. Yoga is beneficial for heart health, concentration and focus, and also to help combat depression.

The Sun Salutation

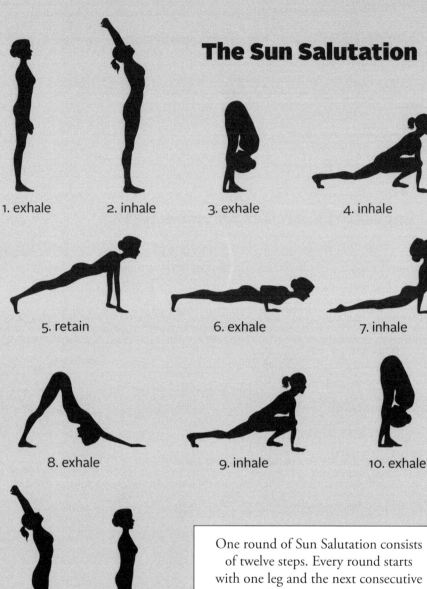

1. exhale

2. inhale

3. exhale

4. inhale

5. retain

6. exhale

7. inhale

8. exhale

9. inhale

10. exhale

11. inhale

12. exhale, inhale and begin again at 1.

One round of Sun Salutation consists of twelve steps. Every round starts with one leg and the next consecutive round is started with the next alternative leg.

One full cycle includes two rounds, one with each leg. Most people recommend 6 cycles each day.

The 12 steps of the Sun Salutation are as follows:

1. Stand straight with the legs together and palms together. Exhale.

2. Stretch the hands above the head and bend the trunk backwards. Then, inhale fully.

3. Bend the body and touch your knees to your forehead. Touch your palms on the floor on either side of your legs. Exhale fully.

4. Kick the right leg back, take the left knee forward, look up and inhale.

5. Push the left leg back and rest only on your palms and toes; keep your body straight from head to toe. Retain.

6. From this position rest the knees on the floor. Leave your palms and toes in place. Rest your chest and forehead on the ground. The buttocks will be raised up. Exhale.

7. Inhale as you raise your head and trunk making the spine concave upwards and straightening your arms without changing the position of your hands and feet.

8. Exhale. Raise your buttocks, push your head down and make a complete arch with your heels touching the ground and palms your palms on the floor.

9. Push the left leg back and rest only on your palms and toes; keep the body straight from head to toe. Inhale.

10. Bring your right foot up next to your left foot between the two hands. Arch the back. Bend the body and touch your knees to your forehead. Touch your palms on the floor on either side of your legs. Exhale fully.

11. Inhale. Stretch the hands above the head and bend the trunk backwards.

12. Stand up with hands along the body and relax. Exhale, inhale, and begin again.

Pilates is a system of exercises designed to improve flexibility, physical strength and enhance mental awareness. It is considered a low impact workout. It is a good choice of exercise for those who experience joint pain or other muscle issues. Pilates strengthens the core of the body. The focus of this type of exercise is on the muscles of the back, stomach, and buttocks. It helps with mind and body coordination. Pilates works with all of the muscles in the body to increase flexibility while strengthening the muscles.

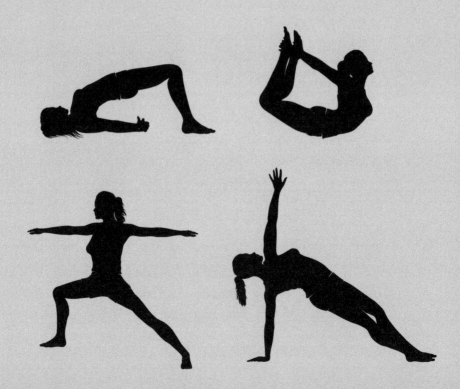

Tai chi is a form of exercise that combines meditation whit gentle body movement. It is a graceful form of exercise often used to combat stress and help with health conditions. This system encourages you to perform a series of movements without pause, your body is in constant motion. There are over 100 possible movements. Tai chi has been known to improve balance, flexibility and muscle strength, relieve chronic pain, increase endurance, and reduce anxiety and depression.

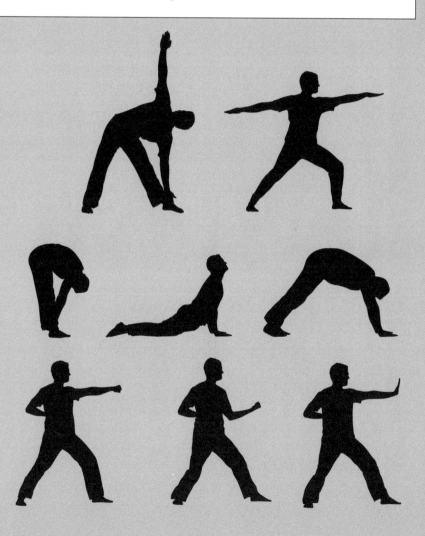

Stretching can increase flexibility and improve range of motion. It can also improve circulation and help to relieve stress. Stretching also provides health benefits, and can reduce muscular soreness and tension, while helping to reduce risk of injury to joints, muscles, and tendons.

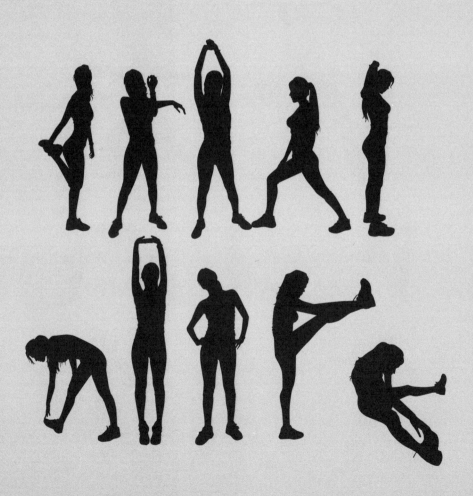

By the numbers

76 billion

In 2000, health care costs associated with physical inactivity were more than $76 billion.

60%

Despite the proven benefits of physical activity, more than 60% of American adults do not get enough physical activity to provide health

5

5 benefits of exercise: Improves your mood. Combats chronic diseases. Helps manage weight. Boosts energy levels. Promotes better sleep.

32.5%

Percent of adults who engaged in regular leisure-time physical activity: 32.5%

25%

According to the Centers for Disease Control and Prevention, more than 25 percent of adults are inactive in their leisure time.

Replace something you already do with something better:

_____

_____

_____

Chapter Eleven
Physical Treatments for Nerve
PROBLEMS

Chiropractic, founded by Dr. Daniel David Palmer in 1895, is a science and art which utilizes the inherent recuperative powers of the body and the relationship between the musculo-skeletal structures and functions of the body, particularly of the spinal column and the nervous system, in the resoration and maintenance of health. The main treatment involves manual therapy. It often includes manipulation of the spine, joints and soft tissues. The therapy is referred to as spinal manipulation or adjustment. The educational requirments for todays Doctor of Chiropractic are among the most stringent of any of the health care professions. People who experience acute and/or chronic pain often seek chiropractic treatment.

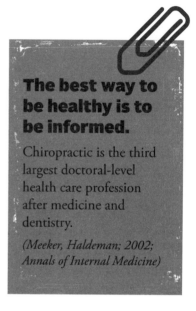

The best way to be healthy is to be informed. Chiropractic is the third largest doctoral-level health care profession after medicine and dentistry.

(Meeker, Haldeman; 2002; Annals of Internal Medicine)

Chiropractors may employ a number of different types of treatment. The most common treatment is often referred to as an adjustment. The practitioner works mainly with the spine to increase the range and quality of motion. Other types of treatment may include electrical nerve stimulation, ultrasound, rehabilitative exercise, heat and ice treatments, dietary supplements, herbs, homeopathic remedies, acupuncture, and counsel about lifestyle factors that may contribute positively or negatively to overall health.

Chiropractors can help with neuropathy and many other nerve related challenges by restoring a balanced communication with the nervous system. Chiropractic may help if a mis-alignment of the spine, jaw, extremities, or skull is causing problems with the messages being sent along the nerves. Chiropractic is often considered a treatment of choice when it comes to nerve related conditions.

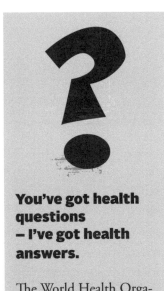

You've got health questions – I've got health answers.

The World Health Organization has determined that acupuncture is an effective therapy for over 200 conditions.

Acupuncture is considered one of the oldest healing practices in the world. This science has been practiced in Asian countries for thousands of years. It is a practice that restores and maintains health through the stimulation of specific points on the body. Acupuncture involves penetrating the skin with thin metallic needles.

Traditional Chinese medicine believes the body has two opposing and inseparable forces, yin and yang. Optimal health is achieved by maintaining a delicate balance between the two. Disease comes from an internal imbalance. If the body is imbalanced it can block the flow of vital energy, qi, along the meridian pathways. Chinese medicine believes that acupuncture can unblock the Qi. Acupuncture is used for prevention or relief of pain and for other health conditions.

The needles used in acupuncture are hair-thin, solid and metallic. Little pain is felt as the needles are inserted. For some people the treatment leaves them feeling energized, others feel relaxed. Acupuncture is thought to be very effective in treating pain. Research suggests that acupuncture may release chemicals that can help numb pain or even block the pain signals that are being sent form the nerves. Studies suggest that acupuncture is an effective form of treatment for peripheral neuropathy and other types of nerve related symptoms. This course of therapy may be a positive choice for those whose condition remains unchanged with current therapy, especially if they are looking for an alternative.

Acupressure is a non-invasive form of acupuncture that uses the fingers to press key points on the surface of the skin to stimulate the body's natural self-curative abilities.

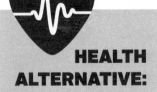

HEALTH ALTERNATIVE:

Reflexology has been practiced for thousands of years by Native Americans, Egyptians, and Mayan and Incan civilizations. Modern reflexology began in the 1930's.

Naturopathic Medicine uses diet exercise and lifestyle changes to enhance the bodies natural ablilty to combat disease. Naturopathic medicine blends the best of modern medical science and traditional natural medical approches. Dr. Benedict Lust was one of the founders of Naturopathic Medicine. There are six principles Naturopathic physicians base their practice on. They are: First, do no harm, Let nature heal, educate patients, identify and treat causes, treat the whole person, and prevent illness.

Reflexology is a non-invasive treatment that involves the use of alternating pressure applied to the reflexes. These reflex points are located on the feet, hands and ears. Reflexology believes that massaging or applying pressure to these points will have a beneficial effect on other parts of the body. Like acupuncture, reflexologists believe that the blockage of Qi can prevent healing. Practitioners relieve stress and pain through manipulation of these reflex points.

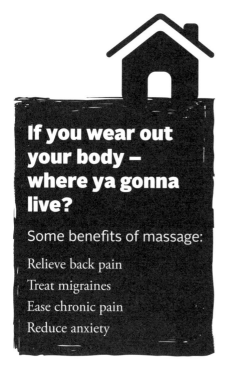

If you wear out your body – where ya gonna live?

Some benefits of massage:

Relieve back pain

Treat migraines

Ease chronic pain

Reduce anxiety

Reflexology is beneficial in aiding circulation. This increase of circulation can be positive and may facilitate a healing of the nerves as circulation increases. The circulation may also help prevent a lack of feeling in the feet. Many have found that the burning pain and numbness that accompanies peripheral neuropathy and other nerve related disorders is decreased when reflexology is done on a consistent basis.

Massage Therapy is one of the oldest healing art forms. Hindus, Persians and Egytians all used massage techniques, and Chinese records document its use over 3,000 years ago. The benefits of massage are

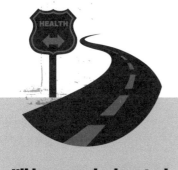

I'll be your designated driver on the highway to health.

3 Tips for Massage Therapy

- Don't eat just before a massage session. Make sure your food has had time to digest.
- Relax your mind and your muscles during the massage session.
- Drink a lot of water after your massage.

varied and far-reaching. Massage can help relieve the stress that accompanies every day living and often leads to disease and illness. It is also beneficial for chronic conditions.

Massage includes soft-tissue manipulation, movement, and repatterning techniques. Therapists may use kneading, compression, stroking tapping, vibration, rocking and pressure. The use of oils, powders, and lotions may also have a role in therapy. The therapy stimulates lymph flow and may enhance immunity. It can stretch tight or atrophied muscles and increase joint flexibility. It improves circulation and reduces spasms and cramping. Massage can release endorphins, which are amino acids that work as natural pain-killers.

Massage therapy can reduce the pain and lessen symptoms associated with neuropathy and other nerve conditions while improving the sense of well-being. Because the therapy promotes blood flow, it increases circulation and the supply of oxygen and nutrients to the sites of pain or discomfort. Massage can also reduce muscle tightness and tension. A common result of massage is the systemic release of endorphins and opiates. This results in pain reduction and a greater sense of well-being.

Prolotherapy is nonsurgical ligament reconstruction. It is considered a treatment for chronic pain. A version of this technique was first used by Hippocrates on soldiers with dislocated or torn shoulder joints. He would stick a hot poker into the joint, and the shoulder would then heal normally. Rather than using a hot poker today, a dextrose solution is injected into the ligament or tendon. This causes a localized inflammation, increasing the blood supply and flow of nutrients, and the tissue is then stimulated to repair itself. Prolotherapy is beneficial when the natural healing process of the body needs a little assistance. It has shown to be effective at eliminating chronic pain.

Hyperbaric Oxygen Therapy is the medical use of 100 percent oxygen at pressures greater than the normal atmosphere. It greatly increases oxygen concentration and improves blood flow to all body tissues. This treatment is administered in a transparent, cylindrical chamber, which varies in size. Treatment usually lasts an hour. If blood flow and oxygen delivery to vital organs is reduced, this therapy should be considered. Hyperbaric Oxygen Therapy is sometimes used to treat specific neurological indications including partial motor or sensory loss.

Biofeedback has been described by the Association for Applied Psychophysiology and Biofeedback as "a process that enables an individual to learn how to change physiological activity for the purposes of improving health and performance. Precise instruments measure physiological activity such as brainwaves, heart function, breathing, muscle activity, and skin temperature. These instruments rapidly and accurately 'feed back' information to the user. The presentation of this information — often in conjunction with changes in thinking, emotions, and behavior — supports desired physiological changes. Over time, these changes can endure without continued use of an instrument."

Several different sensor modalities are used. An electromyography uses surface electrodes to detect muscle action. EMG biofeedback is used when treating chronic pain. A feedback thermometer detects skin temperature. This thermometer is usually attached to a finger or toe. It measures heating and cooling. This modality is also used for chronic pain. A photoplethysmograph measures relative blood flow. It is used to supplement temperature biofeedback when treating chronic pain. Through scientific research, biofeedback has been proven efficacious in dealing with chronic pain.

Biofeedback can help teach you how to control functions within your body that are normally involuntary —for example, your blood pressure or heart rate. It can teach you to relax your muscles and reduce tension, and this may help with relieving pain.

Physical Therapy is a health care profession that provides treatment to help promote maximum movement and function. This profession focuses on improving health for those who are aging, have been injured, or are recovering from surgery. Treatment is also given with relation to disease or environmental factors. Ultrasound, electrical nerve stimulation, and exercise rehabilitation are all courses of treatment that might be used with physical therapy. Another common form of treatment by physical therapists is Cold and Hot Therapy.

Cold and Heat Therapy has long been used for pain and discomfort. These methods can be used individually or alternating, and are two of the most common types of non-invasive therapies. Heat therapy draws blood into the target tissues of pain. This increased blood flow delivers nutrients and oxygen to these areas. Heat is known for its ability to relieve pain and decrease muscle spasm. Cold therapy slows circulation to the area. This reduces inflammation and can also decrease muscle spasm and relieve pain. Cold therapy should be used for less than 20 minutes in most areas of the body

Hot and cold therapy has been used since as early as 1918. This therapy is thought to control the pain level and soreness of the area. Therapy should only last 10-20 minutes. Extensive cold can cause nerve damage, and too much heat may cause burns. Hot and cold therapy has been known to reduce the pain and discomfort of neuropathy.

Antigravity Inversion Therapy

Inversion therapy refers to the technique of treating spinal or nerve conditions through mitigation of gravitational effects, thereby reducing the vertebrae and the discs compression. This allows the ligaments and the muscles surrounding the spine to rest. The devices used for performing this may include hanging upside down from your ankles or pelvis.

Inversion therapy has been used since 400 BC when Hippocrates, the Father of Medicine, strung up a patient on a ladder with ropes and pulleys and allowed gravity to do its work (way before Newton studied gravity force). The concept of inversion was not widely recognized in the United States, however, until Dr. Robert Martin (a California osteopath, chiropractor and medical doctor) introduced the Gravity Guidance System in the 1960's. This revolutionary concept addressed the effects of gravity on the human body, the simple solution of inversion therapy, and the resulting benefits. Inversion tables and traction products have helped many thousands of people

Other Treatment Options to Consider

Besides methods of treating nerve related symptoms, there are certain products that can help alleviate or relieve symptoms associated with nerve disorders.

Special Shoes

One of they symptoms of neuropathy is numbness that can create an insensitivity or a loss of ability to feel heat, cold, and pain. Sometimes a person who suffers from neuropathy will develop minor blisters, cuts or sores that they may not be aware of. It is also common for neuropathy to cause deformities such as hammertoes, bunions and charcot foot.

Your body didn't come with an owner's manual, so I'm here for you.

- 75% of Americans will suffer from some kind of foot problem in their lives.
- Up to 80% of people will suffer from lower back pain at some point in their lives.

One of the ways to guard against this problem is to wear shoes specifically made to protect the feet. This can be harder than it sounds, because many people who suffer from neuropathy often buy shoes that harm their feet. This is due to the fact that neuropathy makes it hard to detect proper shoe size or shape because of the loss of feeling or sensation in the foot. Shoes should extend ½ to ¾ inch beyond the longest toe. The shoes should reduce irritation from walking, be wide and breathable, have soft seamless materials and added toe room. They should be reliable and help to prevent risk of foot injury, should cushion while providing support, and should be made to evenly distribute body weight across the entire foot so that painful pressure points are avoided.

Z coil Shoes are a footware that has been engineered to relieve foot, leg and back pain. These shoes have a shock-absorbing design and can distribute pressure more evenly across the foot. The coil helps to provide less impact for the foot. The footwear protects the foot from injury by providing thick cushioning and padded insoles. They also contain a built-in orthotic.

Orthotics

Orthotics are insoles or shoe inserts worn for the purpose of restoring natural foot function. Over 70 percent of the population suffers from over-pronation, which is when the arches drop and the feet and ankles roll inwards while walking. Orthotic insoles correct this over-pronation and can help realign the foot and anklebones to a healthier position. Because of this ability, orthotics can help reduce or eliminate many aches and pains.

Orthotics can encourage lower extremity biomechanics, while preventing tissue breakdown. They can also absorb shock and help to prevent pressure sores. Emphasis should be placed on relieving pressure areas of both present and potential breakdown. In those who suffer from neuropathy, the goal of the orthotic design should be to provide shock absorption, distribute pressure and reduce high stress areas.

Pronex Cervical Traction

Pronex Cervical Traction is a device that places the patient in a posturally correct position that can allow the body to truly relax. Our common day to day activities can be overwhelming, and often much of our day is spent sitting sedentary as we work. The effects of this can lead to changes in our posture and muscular imbalance leading to nerve related disorders.. Headaches, decreased mobility, and upper extremity sensory symptoms are all side effects of this lifestyle. The Pronex Cervical Traction device helps provide a reduction in muscle tension-related discomfort.

The device provides a gentle controlled stretch to the muscles of the neck and may bring relief of muscle tension and nerve related symptoms. Pronex can be utilized in a professional setting or at-home.

Magnet Therapy

Magnetic fields have been shown to have an effect on living tissue for decades. Plants have been shown to have an improved growth rate when raised in a magnetic field. More recently, doctors and physical therapists have used either static or fluctuating magnetic fields to aid in pain management.

Chapter Twelve

CONCLUSION

Congratulations, you now know more about how to safely, effectively and inexpensively manage and heal nerve related health challenges as a result of reading 'Secret Nerve Cures' than most trained healthcare providers.

The notion of being pain or symptoms free and completely functional may seem unobtainable to someone suffering with either acute or chronic health challenges. As foreign and illogical as it may sound, experiencing pain or some other symptom can be both friend and foe.

Nerves protect our precious health much like idiot lights serve as warnings within the dashboards of automobiles. In the case of our preferred form of transportation, be it car, truck, or motorcycle, if we ignore warning signals such as low oil or water levels, severe damage to an automobile engine may occur. It would be ill advised and costly to ignore an automobile warning light or attempt to cover it up with a brush and paint. Yet in the case of a bodily sign or symptom such as pain or some other type of discomfort, we've been conditioned to merely cover up warning signal or signs with risky side effect laden pharmaceuticals without regard to their intended meaning or cause.

Yes, OTC (over-the-counter) or prescription drugs are sometimes necessary. However, conservative, non-toxic, safe and effective natural approaches should be considered first in most instances.

Having been endowed with nerves by our Devine creator, the human body is able to sense pain and pleasure, learn from mistakes, and adapt within the environment we live. The human body is remarkably resilient and capable of self repair. That is, of course, as long as we're able to remove or reduce that which may be interfering with our ability to do so. Interference to our innate healing process may occur in a number of ways including, but not limited to nerve supply impedance in the form of irritation or inflammation secondary to spinal misalignments called subluxations. Additionally, nutritional deficiencies, psychological stress as well as environmental and lifestyle interference can play a role.

In over three decades of experience as a doctor and radio talk show host, the people I've been honored to serve have taught me many lessons about the miraculous healing resolve of the human body and mind. I sincerely hope you have found the information and observations in this book to be insightful. You should now have a much broader view and understanding with respect to the many possibilities to help resolve nerve related challenges….naturally!

My best wishes for your abundant health and happiness.

Dr. Bob Martin

Companies I recommend

American Health (Ester-C) – 1-866-646-8576 or
www.americanhealthus.com

Dr. Ohhira's Probiotics 12 Plus – 1-800-430-6180 or
drohhiraprobiotics.com.

EuroPharma/Terry Naturally (Curamin) – 1-877-575-5155 or
www.europharmausa.com

LifeTime (vitamins and protein powders) – 1-800-333-6168 or
www.lifetimevitamins.com

KAL (vitamins, minerals, herbs) – 1-800-669-8877 or
www.nutraceutical.com

NaturalCare (herbal, vitamin, homeopathic formulations)
– 1-800-475-9811 www.enaturalcare.com

New Vitality (vitamins, herbs, minerals, skin care, pet products)
– 1-800-764-7482 www.newvitality.com

Nordic Naturals – (Ultimate Omega) – 1-800-787-7208 or
www.nordicnaturals.com

Nutritional Testing Services – 1-800-606-8822 or
www.nutritionaltest.com.

Quincy Bioscience (Prevagen) – 1-888-814-0814 or
www.quincybioscience.com

Solaray (vitamins, minerals, herbs) – 1-800-669-8877 or
www.nutraceutical.com

Tahiti Trader (Noni Juice) - 800-842-5309 or
www.tahititrader.com

Vitamin Research Products – 1-888-578-5111 or
www.vrp.com

Wakunaga (Kyolic – Aged Garlic Extract) – 1-800-421-2998 or
www.kyolic.com

Xlear (Xylitol products) – 1-877-599-5327 or
www.xlear.com

Glossary of Scientific Terms

Antioxidant: an organic substance or enzyme capable of counteracting the damaging effects of oxidation.

Autoimmune disease: a disease that results from a disordered immune reaction when antibodies are used against one's own tissues.

Autonomic Nerves: The part of the nervous system that controls involuntary actions like blood pressure, heart rate, and digestion.

Botanicals: a medicinal preparation derived from part of a plant including leaves, bark, berries or roots.

Central Nervous System: Consists of the brain and spinal cord, and coordinates the activity of the entire nervous system.

Cholinesterase: An enzyme found in blood plasma that hydrolyzes choline esters.

DHEA (dehydroepiandrosterone): a compound secreted by the adrenal glands, which is an intermediate in the biosynthesis of testosterone and estrogens.

Diazepam: A prescribed drug used for alleviation of anxiety and tension, as a muscle relaxant, as a hypnotic, and an anticonvulsant.

Electrochemical impulses: All neurons transmit information in the form of electrochemical reactions. These nerve impulses travel along the nerve fiber to send signals. Impulses involve the movement of electrically charged chemical ions.

Endocrine disorders: Disorders that are often complex, which can involve either hyposecretion or hypersecretion of the endocrine gland.

Fluoroquinolone: A broad spectrum antibiotic derived from quinolone compounds.

Hyperbaric Oxygen Therapy: The administration of oxygen in a chamber. This therapy has various biochemical, cellular and physiologic benefits.

Infectious mononucleosis: A contagious illness caused by the Epstein-Barr virus, which can affect the lymph nodes, liver, and oral cavity.

Morphine: An alkaloid extracted from opium, which can be used in medicine as a light anesthetic, an analgesic, or a sedative.

Motor Nerve: a nerve that stimulates muscle contraction.

Metabolic disorders: any pathophysiologic dysfunction that results in a loss of metabolic control affecting internal equilibrium.

Multidimensional: involving several dimensions.

Neuralgia: Sharp pain which is often severe, extending along a nerve or group of nerves.

Neuroleptic: a major tranquillizer often used in the treatment of psychoses. Reduces the intensity of nerve function.

Neuropathic: Pertains to neuropathy, and is used to describe the nature of nervous disease.

Neuropathy: Any disorder or disease of the nerves.

Oxycodone: A narcotic related to codeine, which can be used as an analgesic and a sedative.

Peripheral Nervous System: Constitutes the nerves outside the central nervous system and includes the spinal nerves, the cranial nerves, and sympathetic and parasympathetic nervous systems.

PH: A measure of the alkalinity or acidity of a solution.

Prebiotic: Prebiotics are non-digestible food ingredients that stimulate the growth and/or activity of bacteria in the digestive system in ways claimed to be beneficial to health.

Probiotic: a preparation that is taken orally to restore beneficial bacteria to the body.

Psychomotor impairment: a reduction of physical movements comprised with a slowing down of thought.

Sensory Nerve: a nerve that passes impulses to the central nervous system.

Subluxation: when spinal bones lose their normal position and motion. This can occur from stress, trauma, or chemical imbalances where communication to and from your brain is interrupted.

Trigeminal Neuralgia: shooting pains of the facial area around one or more branches of the trigeminal nerve.

Glossary of Professional Organizations:

Activator Methods International, Ltd.

2950 N. Seventh Street, Suite 200

Phoenix, Arizona 85014

ofc 602-224-0220

fax 602-224-0230

toll free 1-800-598-0224

American Academy of Pain Management

www.aapainmanage.org

American Association of Naturopathic Physicians (AANP)

3201 New Mexico Avenue, NW, Suite 350

Washington, DC 20016

Phone: 202-895-1392 – 866-538-2267

Website: www.naturopathic.org

American Chiropractic Association

1701 Clarendon Boulevard

Arlington, VA 22209

Phone: 703-276-8800

Fax: 703-243-2593

American Clinical Board of Nutrition

6855 Browntown Road

Front Royal, VA 22630

540-635-8844/Fax 540-635-3669

www.acbn.org

American College for Advancement in Medicine (ACAM)

23121 Verdugo Drive, Suite 204

Laguna Hills, CA 92653

Phone: 949—583-7666 – 800-532-3688

Fax: 949-455-9679

Email: info@acam.org

Website: www.acam.org

American Holistic Medicine Association

4101 Lake Boone Trail, Suite 201

Raleigh, NC 27607

Phone: 919-787-5146

American Massage and therapy Association

152 West Wisconsin Ave.

Milwaukee, WI 53203

Association for Applied Psychophysiology and Biofeedback

10200 W. 44th Avenue, Suite 304

Wheat Ridge, CO 80033-2840

Phone 303-422-8436

Celiac Disease Foundation

13251 Ventura Boulevard, Suite 1

Studio city, Ca 91604-1838

Phone: 818-990-2354

Website: http://www.celiac.org

Fibromyalgia Network
PO box 31750
Tucson, AZ 85751
Phone: 800-853-2929
Website: http://www.fmnetnews.com

FFTF, LLC
7 Benmere Road
Glen Burnie, MD 21060
Email: office@endfatigue.com
Phone: 410-573-5389
Fax: 410-590-3047
Website: www.endfatigue.com

International Academy of Medical Acupuncture Inc.
Phone: 800-327-1113
Website: www.IAMA.edu

International and American Associations of Clinical Nutritionists (IAACN)
15280 Addison Road, Suite 130
Addison, TX 75001
Phone: 972-407-9089
Website: www.iaacn.org

International Foundation for Homeopathy
2366 Eastlake Ave. E., Suite 301
Seattle WA 98102
Phone: 206-324-8230

International Yoga Institute

227 west 13th Street

New York, NY 10011

National Center for Complementary and Alternative Medicine

9000 Rockville Pike

Bethesda, MD 20892

Website: www.nccam.nih.gov

National Center for Homeopathy

801 North Fairfax Street, Suite 306

Alexandria, VA 22314

Phone: 703-548-7790

National Certification Commission for Acupuncture and Oriental Medicine (NCCAOM)

76 South Laura Street, suite 1290

Jacksonville, FL 32202

Phone: 904-598-1005

National Chronic Pain Outreach Association

7979 Old Georgetown Road, Suite 100

Bethesda, MD 20814

Phone: 301-652-4948

Chronic Fatigue & Fibromyalgia

Dr. Jacob Teitelbaum

The National Foundation for the Treatment of Pain

1714 white Oak Drive

Houston, TX 77009

Phone: 713-862-9332

Website: www.paincare.org

Tai Chi society

1047 Amsterdam Ave.

New York, NY 10025

Phone: 212-865-6096

Nutritional Testing Services

Invites you to:

STOP GUESSING.... about which nutritional supplement(s) is best for you. Our services provide a much needed professional roadmap defining where to begin and what to do. Over time you'll save money and have peace-of-mind in knowing you're taking the correct supplements to meet your individual nutritional needs.

Objective science based testing for nutritional imbalances or deficiencies is not merely for people who are currently experiencing some type of pain, discomfort, health crisis, concern or symptom(s), but also for health prevention and preservation.

Nutritional testing can be invaluable even for healthy people because almost all of us are born with inherited genetic weaknesses causing us to be more prone to certain illnesses. The old adage, 'don't fix if it isn't broken' might be ok for some things, however when it comes to our precious health it can prove to be very costly if not outright deadly.

Available tests and analysis in the privacy of your own home:

Comprehensive Digestive Test

The Comprehensive Digestive Test is a group of 15 to 22 tests performed via saliva and stool samples, revealing valuable information about your gastrointestinal and overall health. The Comprehensive Digestive Test evaluates digestion efficiency, the presence of hidden yeast or bacterial infections, food allergies, specific enzyme ranges, intestinal flora balance, the presence of parasites and ova, intestinal immune function, toxic reactions to a certain food group, the presence of occult blood, fecal pH and others. Think of the time and money you spend planning menus, shopping for food, preparing meals and buying vitamin supplements. How do you know if you're getting the most from your food or supplements? Could your diet and lifestyle be causing other problems in your body that you're not aware of?

With changes in the modern American diet, gastrointestinal disorders have become increasingly prevalent. One recent study reported that over a period of three months, gastrointestinal symptoms were experienced in over 70% of American households. Often poor digestion and absorption, abnormal intestinal flora, parasitic infections, yeast and fungus overgrowth, harmful bacteria, as well as many chronic illnesses and symptoms, lie at the root of many common digestive system complaints

The Comprehensive Digestive Test provides critical information through a non-invasive assessment panel for evaluating the health status of your digestive tract. Through a number of important biomarkers tests, the Comprehensive Digestive Test helps pinpoint imbalances, provides clues about current symptoms, and warns of potential health problems. A personalized treatment program can be suggested and easily applied, greatly increasing your chances of responding naturally.

What can a Comprehensive Digestive Test tell me?
Think of your body as a finely tuned engine, and food as its fuel. If

you aren't completely digesting foods and absorbing nutrients, then you're not adequately fueling your body. The lack of adequate fuel or the inability to use it properly can lead to a variety of health problems such as poor digestion or imbalances in your intestinal flora which can result in many illnesses including annoying gastrointestinal complaints such as chronic constipation, diarrhea, abdominal discomfort, or even more serious illnesses which may appear to be unrelated to digestion, such as asthma, skin problems, arthritis, fatigue, headaches, yeast infections, hemorrhoids, fibromyalgia, allergies, a weakened immune system and the list goes on and on.

Gastrointestinal health is the goal: For proper gastrointestinal health, your body must carefully coordinate the breakdown, absorption and elimination of food. Bacteria must be in proper balance, and immune function must be adequate. The Comprehensive Digestive Test provides an easy to understand and effective evaluation of how well your gastrointestinal tract functions and performs.

Stool and Saliva sample collection is a convenient, non-invasive and stress-free procedure, and is cost-effective since samples can easily be collected at home or work. Instructions are simple and easy to follow.

Mineral & Toxic Metal Test

The average American will be exposed to over 100,000 toxic chemicals in a lifetime, according to estimates. With the enormous amounts of toxic metals in the environment and widespread nutrient mineral insufficiencies, assessing imbalances, deficiencies and excesses is very important. A Mineral and Toxic Metal Test and Analysis via hair analysis is an accurate method of evaluating mineral and heavy metal imbalances and toxicities. The Mineral and Toxic Metal Test provides an assessment of long-term toxic element exposure. Toxic metals measured for in this test include lead, mercury, cadmium, arsenic, aluminum and others. Additionally, nutrient mineral levels are measured including calcium, magnesium, sodium, potassium, iron, copper, manganese zinc and others. It's non-invasive, inexpensive and allows for investigation of nutrient/toxin interactions.

Hair collection is a convenient, non-invasive, stress-free procedure, and is cost-effective since samples can easily be collected at home or work. Instructions are simple and easy to follow.

Nutritional Blood Analysis

How many times have you been to a doctor because you weren't feeling well only to be told after a series of blood tests, that everything is normal? Don't worry, you're not alone! It happens to millions of people every day. Allopathic (MD) doctors, and the lab tests they use are best at identifying disease that is already established. The good news is that subtle changes can be detected and identified earlier using sophisticated blood lab analysis. The Comprehensive Nutritional Blood Analysis can help determine subtle abnormal shifts in blood tests ranges in advance of serious events. Additionally, if you have current health concerns or challenges, you'll receive a detailed written nutrition regimen to help rebalance any discovered nutritional deficiencies or imbalances.

You may choose to use a current and complete blood lab panel to obtain a Comprehensive Nutritional Blood Analysis or obtain a new panel via our service.

You will receive a detailed written report of nutritional and lifestyle findings and recommendations by a doctor and board certified Clinical Nutritionist via U.S. Priority Mail.

Hormone Level test

Research shows that sex hormones play a key role in shaping the course of health in both men and women. Hormones are powerful substances that control many functions throughout the body. Excess or deficiency creates problems in physical, mental or emotional health. Hormone saliva testing and analysis is considered by many health experts to be the most accurate and reliable way to measure true body hormone levels. Saliva hormone collection is a convenient, non-invasive, and stress-free procedure, and is cost-effective since samples can easily be collected at home or work. Instructions are simple and easy to follow.

Please choose from any of our Nutritional Test and Analysis Offerings. For further information or to order one or more of the above, please call Nutritional Testing Services at 1-800-606-8822 or www.nutritionaltest.com.

Objective Tests:

C-reactive protein

C-reactive protein is produced by the liver. The level of CRP in blood rises when there is inflammation in the body.

Musculoskelatal Ultrasound Imaging

Musculoskeletal ultrasound imaging enables physicians to document and evaluate pathological soft tissue densities. Through the use of high-frequency, high-resolution transducers, excellent quality images of soft tissue are provided. These tests provide important information for determining the cause of musculoskeletal symptoms/disorders.

Somatosensory and Dermatomal Evoked Potential Studies

Evoked potential studies evaluate the central nervous system by examining sensory tracts in the spinal cord connecting the extremities to the brain. Studies detect physiological impairment through proximal parts of peripheral nerves, spinal nerve roots, the spinal cord, and the brainstem.

Blood Glucose Test – a fasting blood test used to detect hyperglycemia (high blood sugar) or hypoglycemia (low blood sugar).

Serum Protein – A total serum protein test measures the total amount of protein in the blood.

Blood Triglycerides - Triglycerides are the fats carried in the blood.

Methylmalonic Acid Test - MMA (urine or blood) - The methylmalonic acid (MMA) test is a sensitive and early indicator of vitamin B12 deficiency at the tissue level. NOTE: Non-MMA blood testing for B-12 deficit is notorious for false findings.

Homocysteine Blood Test – A homocysteine test determines if a person has B12 or folate deficiency. The homocysteine concentration may be elevated before B12 and folate tests are abnormal.

Thermography

This procedure measures the temperature on the skin surface to locate inflammation of muscles and soft tissues. A special camera takes pictures, which reflect the different temperatures by displaying a range of colors on film. Thermography has been used to pinpoint spinal nerve and muscle stress. Thermography remains the only method available for visualizing pain and inflammation. This safe, cost effective and risk free evaluation is a very useful adjunctive procedure to other diagnostic tools.

Nerve Conduction Velocity

Similar to testing current flow in a wire, nerve conduction velocity test (NCV) is an electrical test, ordered by your doctor, used to detect abnormal nerve conditions. It is usually ordered to diagnose or evaluate a nerve injury in a person who has weakness or numbness in the arms or legs. It also helps to discover how severe the condition is and how a nerve is responding to injury or to treatment. A healthy nerve will transmit the signal faster and stronger than a sick nerve.

The EMG (Electromyogram) Test

An EMG (electromyogram) may be ordered to see if you have a pinched nerve in the back or the neck. If you have tingling or numbness in your arms or legs, an EMG may also show if you have nerve pressure there. The EMG measures the electrical activity in muscles. Muscles normally receive constant electrical signals from healthy nerves.

Reference sites used

www.mayoclinic.com

www.iom.edu

www.ana-jana.org

www.about.com

www.wikipedia.com

http://ods.od.nih.gov

www.ccjm.org

www.merck.com

www.ninds.nih.gov

www.emedicehealth.com

www.diabetes.org

www.nervedisorders.com

www.ncbi.nlm.nih.gov

www.neuropathy.org

http://jama.ama-assn.org

www.ama-assn.org

www.fda.gov

http://medind.nic.in/

www.oandp.org

www.parentsasteachers.org

www.safefood.org

www.naturalnews.com

www.webmd.com

- **Research on adverse side effects of drugs:**

Neuropathy Drugs Increase Suicide Risk BMJ. 2007 Jul 14;335(7610):87. Epub 2007 Jun 11. The FDA performed the study. Results showed there was twice the risk of suicidal behavior for those using the anti-epileptic drugs. The medications studied were:

Carbamazepine (marketed as Carbatrol, Equetro, Tegretol, Tegretol XR)

Felbamate (marketed as Felbatol)

Gabapentin (marketed as Neurontin)

Lamotrigine (marketed as Lamictal)

Levetiracetam (marketed as Keppra)

Oxcarbazepine (marketed as Trileptal)

Pregabalin (marketed as Lyrica)

Tiagabine (marketed as Gabitril)

Topiramate (marketed as Topamax)

Valproate (marketed as Depakote, Depakote ER, Depakene, Depacon)

Zonisamide (marketed as Zonegran)

- **Diabetes Studies:**

Diabetes. 1997 Sep;46 Suppl 2:S62-6. Alpha-lipoic acid in the treatment of diabetic peripheral and cardiac autonomic neuropathy. Ziegler D, Gries FA.

Effects of 3-week oral treatment with the antioxidant thioctic acid (alpha-lipoic acid) in symptomatic diabetic polyneuropathy. Ruhnau KJ, Meissner HP, Finn JR, Reljanovic M, Lobisch M, Schütte K, Nehrdich D, Tritschler HJ, Mehnert H, Ziegler D. PMID: 10656234 [PubMed - indexed for MEDLINE] Free Radic Biol Med. 1999 Aug;27(3-4):309-14. Diabet Med. 1999 Dec;16(12):1040-3.

Oral administration of RAC-alpha-lipoic acid modulates insulin sensitivity in patients with type-2 diabetes mellitus: a placebo-controlled pilot trial. Jacob S, Ruus P, Hermann R, Tritschler HJ, Maerker E, Renn W, Augustin HJ, Dietze GJ, Rett K. Hypertension and Diabetes Research Unit, Max Grundig Clinic, Bühl and City Hospital, Baden-Baden, Germany. snjacob@med.uni-tuebingen.de Treat Endocrinol. 2004;3(3):173-89.

Thioctic acid for patients with symptomatic diabetic polyneuropathy: a critical review. Ziegler D. German Diabetes Clinic, German Diabetes Research Institute, Leibniz Institute at the Heinrich Heine University, Düsseldorf, Germany. dan.ziegler@ddfi.uni-duesseldorf. de PMID: 16026113 [PubMed - indexed for MEDLINE]Diabetes. 2009 Jul;58(7):1634-40. Epub 2009 May 1.

Elevated triglycerides correlate with progression of diabetic neuropathy. Wiggin TD, Sullivan KA, Pop-Busui R, Amato A, Sima AA, Feldman EL. Department of Neurology, University of Michigan, Ann Arbor, MI, USA. PMID: 19411614 [PubMed - indexed for MEDLINE]PMCID: PMC2699859 [Available on 2010/7/1]Free Article Diabet Med. 2000 Apr;17(4):259-68.

Sorbitol and myo-inositol levels and morphology of sural nerve in relation to peripheral nerve function and clinical neuropathy in men with diabetic, impaired, and normal glucose tolerance. Sundkvist G, Dahlin LB, Nilsson H, Eriksson KF, Lindgärde F, Rosén I, Lattimer SA, Sima AA, Sullivan K, Greene DA. Department of Endocrinology, University of Lund, Malmö University Hospital, Sweden. goran.

sundkvist@endo.mas.lu.se PMID: 10821291 [Pubmed - indexed for MEDLINE]

Early peripheral nerve abnormalities in impaired glucose tolerance. Cappellari A, Airaghi L, Capra R, Ciammola A, Branchi A, Levi Minzi G, Bresolin N. Service of Clinical Neurophysiology, Dino Ferrari Centre, Department of Neurological Sciences, IRCCS Ospedale Maggiore di Milano and University of Milan, Milan, Italy. albertocapp@yahoo.it PMID: 16083148 [PubMed - indexed for MEDLINE]

Effects of treatments for symptoms of painful diabetic neuropathy: systematic review. Wong MC, Chung JW, Wong TK. Nursing Services Division, United Christian Hospital, 130 Hip Wo Street, Hong Kong. wongmc0829@yahoo.com.hk Evid Based Med. 2008 Feb;13(1):21. ACP J Club. 2008 Jan-Feb;148(1):2. J Fam Pract. 2007 Oct;56(10):793. PMID: 17562735 [PubMed - indexed for MEDLINE]PMCID: PMC1914460Free PMC Article

• HIV/AIDS Studies
Symptom management and self-care for peripheral neuropathy in HIV/AIDS. AIDS Care. 2007 Feb;19(2):179-89. Nicholas PK, Kemppainen JK, Canaval GE, Corless IB, Sefcik EF, Nokes KM, Bain CA, Kirksey KM, Eller LS, Dole PJ, Hamilton MJ, Coleman CL, Holzemer WL, Reynolds NR, Portillo CJ, Bunch EH, Wantland DJ, Voss J, Phillips R, Tsai YF, Mendez MR, Lindgren TG, Davis SM, Gallagher DM. PMID: 17364396 [PubMed - indexed for MEDLINE]

- **Studies on Exercise:**

Yoga Reduces Inflammation Implicated in Stress and Aging. Posted on 2010-01-15 06:00:00 in Alternative Medicine | Inflammation | Stress | Janice K. Kiecolt-Glaser, Lisa Christian, Heather Preston, Carrie R. Houts, William B. Malarkey, Charles F. Emery, Ronald Glaser. "Stress, Inflammation, and Yoga Practice." Psychosom Med 2010 : PSY.0b013e3181cb9377v1.

Stress, Inflammation, and Yoga Practice. Janice K. Kiecolt-Glaser , PhD, Lisa Christian , PhD, Heather Preston , BA, Carrie R. Houts, MS, William B. Malarkey , MD, Charles F. Emery , PhD, Ronald Glaser, PhD

- **Studies on Nutrition, Nutraceuticals, and healthy foods:**

External antirheumatic and antineuralgic herbal remedies in the traditional medicine of north-eastern Italy. J Ethnopharmacol. 1982 Sep;6(2):161-90. Cappelletti EM, Trevisan R, Caniato R.PMID: 6982378 [PubMed - indexed for MEDLINE]

An ethnobotanical study of traditional anti-inflammatory plants used by the Lohit community of Arunachal Pradesh, India. J Ethnopharmacol. 2009 Sep 7;125(2):234-45. Epub 2009 Jul 14. Namsa ND, Tag H, Mandal M, Kalita P, Das AK.Department of PMID: 19607898 [PubMed - indexed for MEDLINE]

- **Acetyl-L-Carnitine Research:**

Protective effect of acetyl-L-carnitine on the apoptotic pathway of peripheral neuropathy. Eur J Neurosci. 2007 Aug;26(4):820-7. Di

Cesare Mannelli L, Ghelardini C, Calvani M, Nicolai R, Mosconi L, Vivoli E, Pacini A, Bartolini A. Department of Preclinical and Clinical Pharmacology, University of Florence, 50139, Florence, Italy. lorenzo. mannelli@unifi.it PMID: 17714181 [PubMed - indexed for MEDLINE]

Acetyl-L-carnitine improves pain, nerve regeneration, and vibratory perception in patients with chronic diabetic neuropathy: an analysis of two randomized placebo-controlled trials. Sima AA, Calvani M, Mehra M, Amato A; Acetyl-L-Carnitine Study Group.Department of Pathology, Wayne State University School of Medicine, Detroit, Michigan 48201, USA. asima@med.wayne.edu PMID: 15616239 [PubMed - indexed for MEDLINE]Free Article

Thioctic acid and acetyl-L-carnitine in the treatment of sciatic pain caused by a herniated disc: a randomized, double-blind, comparative study. Clin Drug Investig. 2008;28(8):495-500. Memeo A, Loiero M. Ortopedia Pediatrica, Istituto Ortopedico Gaetano Pini, Milan, Italy. antoniomemeo@katamail.com PMID: 18598095 [PubMed - indexed for MEDLINE]

- **Methyl B12 Research:**

Regeneration of Motor Nerve Terminals with Methyl B12 Methylcobalamine (methyl-B12) Promotes Regeneration of Motor Nerve Terminals Degenerating in anterior gracile muscle of gracile axonal dystrophy (GAD) mutant mouse Yamazaki K Oda K Endo C Kikuchi T Wakabayashi T, Neurosci Lett (1994 Mar 28) 170(1):195-7

Benfotiamine and Improvement in Nerve Conduction VelocityA
Benfotiamine-vitamin B Combination in Treatment of Diabetic
Polyneuropathy Stracke H, Lindemann A, Federlin K. Third Medical
Department, University of Giessen, Germany. Exp Clin Endocrinol
Diabetes. 1996;104(4):311-6.

Effectiveness of Different Benfotiamine Dosage Regimens in the
Treatment of Painful Diabetic Neuropathy Winkler G, Pal B, Nagy-
beganyi E, Ory I, Porochnavec M, Kempler P. 2nd Department of
Internal Medicine, Municipal St. John's Hospital, Budapest, Hun-
gary. Arzneimittelforschung. 1999 Mar;49(3):220-4. Abstract

• Research for Alternative Methods:
Peripheral neuropathy: pathogenic mechanisms and alternative
therapies. Altern Med Rev. 2006 Dec;11(4):294-329. Head KA.
Thorne Research, Inc., PO Box 25, Dover, ID 83825, USA. PMID:
17176168 [PubMed - indexed for MEDLINE]Free Article

Index

bloating, 38, 41, 67
blueberries, 104
blurred vision, 37, 70
behavioral, 29
Bell's Palsy, 22, 90
 symptoms of, 22
 care of, 22
black elderberry extract, 33
blisters, 33
blood flow, 80, 146, 148
Blood Glucose Test, 177
blood pressure, 15, 26
blood tests, 41
Blood Triglycerides, 177
blood vessels, 89
bone degeneration, 14
boswellia, 114
botanical oils, 81, 111
botanical plants, 106
 list of, 106
botanical products, 96, 114
botanical remedies, 23, 24 25, 26, 27, 28, 31, 34, 37,
brain, 27, 28, 29, 39, 40, 52, 90, 125
 electrical activity, 58
 healthy brain function, 29
 neurons, 58
 swelling, 56
brain damage, 28. 67
 causes of, 28
 symptoms of, 28
breathing, 14, 27
Bristol Homeopathic Hospital, 86
bronchospasm, 59
bruising, 40, 116
burning, 13, 21, 24, 25, 26, 27, 30, 31, 34, 35, 36, 45, 58, 86, 87, 88, 91, 99

C

Calamine Lotion, 33
calcarea carbonica, 89
calcium, 28, 29, 43
calcium oxide, 90
calf, 34, 89
chamomile, 115
camphor, 115
cancer, 16, 27, 35, 36, 55
capsaicin, 33, 80, 111
capsicum, 113
cardiac disease, 116

carpal tunnel syndrome, 21, 23, 25, 32
 symptoms of, 23
 care of, 23
carbon monoxide, 55, 56
 effects of, 56
cardiac autonomic nerve dysfunction, 99
causticum, 90
celia disease, 35
celiac disease, 41
 statistics on, 42
 symptoms of, 41
cells, 52
central nervous system, 3, 38, 54, 56, 87, 98, 101
Centers for Disease Control and Prevention, 55
chemicals, 45, 52
chemotherapy, 25, 30, 36
chest pain, 26, 59
chickenpox, 33
chills, 45
chiropractic, 141-142
chloroquine, 48
cholesterol lowering foods, 102
cholinesterase, 56
chronic disease, 95, 98
chronic illness, 26
 causes of, 29
 neurological, 57
chronic pain, 36, 37, 38, 103, 113, 141, 147
cimetidine, 48
cimicifuga racemosa, 85
cisplatin, 48
coccyx, 91
cognitive, 29
colchicine, 48
cold and heat therapy, 148
Comprehensive Digestive Test, 171-172
clocynth, 86
colocynthis, 86
Complex Regional Pain Syndrome, 25, 36
 symptoms of, 36
Comprehensive Digestive Test, 38, 41, 42
Comprehensive Nutritional Analysis, 38, 40, 42, 43
confusion, 66, 71
consciousness, loss of, 56
constipation, 26, 70
control blood sugar levels, 80

coordination, 39, 54, 56
    lack of, 47, 71
costs of nervous system conditions, 5
corboxyhemoglobin, 56
cough, 47, 48
cramps, 30, 89, 91, 123, 145
    leg cramps, 44
    symptoms of, 30
C-reactive protein blood test, 45, 177
Crohn's disease, 102
cubital tunnel syndrome, 23
curcumin, 103
cyanide, 55
cytokines, 102

D

death, 56
decreased energy, 38
degenerative neurological illness, 28
devil's claw, 115
depression, 44, 48, 66
dextrose solution, 146
DHEA(dehydroepiandrosterone), 40, 44
diabetes, 15, 16, 24, 25, 30, 32, 35, 36, 27, 58, 71, 105
    symptoms,of, 37
    care of, 37
    Type 1 diabetes, 37
    Type 2 Diabetes, 37, 67, 99
diabetes studies, 180
diabetic neuropathy, 24, 100-102, 123, 124
    symptoms of, 24
    care of, 24
diabetic peripheral neuropathy, 99
diagnosing nerve pain, 15-17
diarrhea, 47, 67
Diazepam, 71
difficulty concentrating, 38
difficulty swallowing, 47
digestion, 26
digestive system, 89
dimethyl sulfoxide, 113
diminished pain perception, 35
diminished thermal perception, 35
discomfort, 65
disease, 53, 55, 83, 84, 88, 98, 145
    management, 65
disulfiram, 48
dizziness, 15, 38, 39, 44, 48, 56, 57, 66, 70, 98

Doctor of Chiropractic, 141
double vision, 39
DPM (Doctor of Pediatric Medicine), 80
Dr. Ohirrah's Probiotics 12 Plus, 107, 159
drawing blood, 36
drooling, 22
drooping eyelid, 22
drowsiness, 56, 59
drug labels, 66
drug therapy, 66
dry eyes, 22, 26
dry mouth, 70
DRX-9000 (specialized form of spinal traction), 43
dull pain, 30
dust, 54
dysfunctional hereditary gene, 28

E

eating right, 79
echinacea, 33
edema, 70
Edison, Thomas, 95
Egypt, 114
Egyptians, 143, 144
electric shocks, 88, 91
electrical nerve stimulation, 141, 147
electrochemical impulses, 4
EMG, 147, 178
emotional, 29
endocrine imbalance, 38
endorphins, 145
enlarged spleen, 42
environmental toxins, 27, 44, 48
enzymes, 96
Epstein Barr, 42
    infection, 42
    symptoms of, 42
    virus
Epstein Barr virus, 42
Erb, John, 60
essential oils, 112
estrogen, 44
eugenol, 112
Europe, 77, 85, 87, 114
EuroPharma, 103, 159
European folk medicine, 85
evening primrose oil, 102
excessive tearing, 22
excitatory neurotransmitter, 58

excitotoxin, 60
Excitotoxins: The Taste that Kills, 57
exercise, 43, 44, 79, 80, 90, 131
exercises for nerve health, 131-137
        statistics on, 137
extreme hunger, 37
extreme sensitivity, 35, 36
eye pain, 22
        damage, 67
eye problems, 58

F

facial hair growth, 44
facial neuralgia, 85
facial pain, 21, 31
facial paralysis, 22
facial tenderness, 38
facial weakness, 22
fainting, 15
fatal, 84
fatigue, 37, 38, 40, 42, 44, 45, 48, 57, 67
fatty acids, 96
FDA, 58, 71
Federation of American Societies for Experimental Biology (FASEB), 58
ferrum phosphoricum, 90
fever, 40, 42, 45, 47, 113
        reducer, 114
fibroblasts, 15
fibrocystic breasts, 44
Fibromyalgia, 25, , 69
        symptoms of, 38
fibrous tissue, 32
fingertips, 34
fish oil, 102
flaky skin, 47
flu-like symptoms, 33, 46
fluid retention, 44
fluoroquinolone, antibiotics, 71
food science, 95
foot, 32
        care, 80
folic acid, 105, 106
fracture, 36
free radicals, 98
frequent infection, 37
fungicides, 56

G

Gandhi, Mahatma, 83
gastrointestinal reaction, 67
gastrointestinal symptoms, 41
gastrointestinal system, 106
general pain, 45
genes, 77
Germany, 83
ginger, 98
Glossary of Professional Organizations, 165
Glossary of Scientific Terms, 161
gliadin, 41
glucosamine and chondroitin, 114
glucose, 99
glucose level, 37, 80
glutamate, 58, 60
gluten, 41
        intolerance, 41
glycyrrhiza glabra (licorice), 116
goto kola, 100
gout, 102-103
Gravity Guidance System, 149
Greece, 114
gunshot wound, 36

H

Hahnemann, Samuel Christian, 83, 90
hair loss, 40, 44
hallucination, 66
hands, 34
HBOT (hyperbaric oxygen therapy), 28
headache, 31, 33, 44, 45, 48, 54, 57, 59, 69, 71, 91, 113, 114, 115, 151
healing affirmations, 81-82
        benefits of affirmations, 81
health alternative, 99
healthcare, 77
heart, 46, 89
heart disease, 55
hemoglobin, 56
heel, 32
hepatitis, 35
herbicides, 48, 56
herbal formulas, 43
herbs, 22, 23, 83, 85, 98, 100, 142
herpes, 47
high blood pressure, 116
Hindus, 144

tumeric, 103
Twain, Mark, 82
twitching, 14, 22, 27, 100

U

ultrasound, 23, 141, 147
United States, 102
University of Wisconsin—Milwaukee, 28
US Food and Drug Administration, 95
US Surgeon General, 55
unusual thirst, 37
urinary symptoms, 39
      frequent urination, 37
urinary tract infection, 44

V

van Gogh, Vincent, 77
velvet antler, 101
vasculitis, 35
verbascum, 88
vertebrae, 148
violent pains, 87
viruses, 77
visceral pain, 86
vision loss, 39, 47, 125
      double, 71
vitamins, 22, 23, 25, 26, 27, 31, 33, 34, 37, 41, 58, 79, 80, 96, 101
      B12, 41, 80, 99
      vitamin B1, 104
      vitamin B-3
      vitamin B 6, 122
      vitamin B9
      vitamin B12, 41, 80, 99, 106, 123
      vitamin C, 103, 107
      vitamin chart, 96-97
      vitamin D, 102, 124
      vitamin therapy, 28
vitamin B complex, 122
      signs of deficiency, 122
vitamin B6 food sources, 122
vitamin B12 food sources, 123
vitamin D, 124
      food sources for, 124
Vitamin Research Products, 160
vomiting, 71

W

Wakanaga Kyolic-Aged Garlic Extract, 33, 160
walnuts, 124, 125
weakness, 27, 41, 44, 54, 58
weakness in limbs, 38, 39, 46
weight fluctuation, 37
weight gain, 70
weight loss, 41, 47
Western culture, 83
whiplash, 31
white blood cell count, 67
white willow bark, 114
wintergreen, 113
World Health Organization, The, 57, 77, 142
wrist pain, 23

X

Xlear, 160

Y

yeast infection, 47
yin and yang, 142
yoga, 131

Z

zingiber officinale (ginger), 115